Improving Trauma and Critical Care Proficiency and Readiness for Air Force Personnel in Critical Medical Specialties

A Pacific Air Forces Perspective

LISA M. HARRINGTON, EDWARD W. CHAN, CARL BERDAHL, MATTHEW WALSH, SEAN MANN, JONAH KUSHNER, SHREYAS BHARADWAJ, MARK TOUKAN, THOMAS GOUGHNOUR

Prepared for the Department of the Air Force
Approved for public release; distribution unlimited

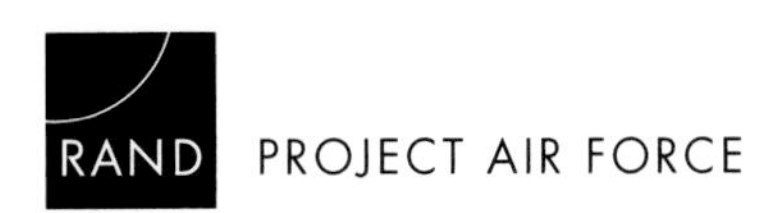

PROJECT AIR FORCE

For more information on this publication, visit **www.rand.org/t/RRA993-1**.

About RAND

Research Integrity

Published by the RAND Corporation, Santa Monica, Calif.

Library of Congress Cataloging-in-Publication Data is available for this publication.

ISBN: 978-1-9774-1085-6

Cover: Marisa Alia-Novobilski/U.S. Air Force.

Limited Print and Electronic Distribution Rights

About This Report

The RAND Corporation's Project AIR FORCE was asked to examine the challenges faced by U.S. Air Force medical personnel in acquiring and maintaining the skills for clinical proficiency and readiness for wartime, especially those in Pacific Air Forces. The goal of this research project was to investigate approaches for increasing readiness and proficiency and to suggest a systematic approach for the Air Force Medical Service to follow when identifying who needs training to maintain readiness, what type of training is needed, and how to consider a portfolio of activities for meeting those needs.

In this report we provide demographics for 14 critical medical Air Force Specialty Codes (AFSCs) selected by the sponsor, review the Air Force's medical readiness requirements for specific AFSCs, and assess the system for monitoring whether medical personnel have met the requirements. We then provide a set of activities and policies that would increase medical personnel readiness that were gathered from meetings with stakeholders and a review of literature. Finally, we discuss an approach for developing a portfolio of readiness building activities applicable across locations and specialties.

This report should be of interest to decisionmakers responsible for policies aimed at ensuring the proficiency of medical personnel in critical specialties, as well as the development and assignment of these medical personnel. More broadly, the research will be of interest to those who study military medical readiness and military manpower and personnel issues.

The research reported here was commissioned by Pacific Air Forces and conducted within the Workforce, Development, and Health Program of RAND Project AIR FORCE as part of a fiscal year 2021 project titled "Effective Approaches to Maintain Currency for High Demand/Low Density Active Duty Medical Fields."

RAND Project AIR FORCE

RAND Project AIR FORCE (PAF), a division of the RAND Corporation, is the Department of the Air Force's (DAF's) federally funded research and development center for studies and analyses, supporting both the United States Air Force and the United States Space Force. PAF provides the DAF with independent analyses of policy alternatives affecting the development, employment, combat readiness, and support of current and future air, space, and cyber forces. Research is conducted in four programs: Strategy and Doctrine; Force Modernization and Employment; Resource Management; and Workforce, Development, and Health. The research reported here was prepared under contract FA7014-16-D-1000.

Additional information about PAF is available on our website:
www.rand.org/paf/

This report documents work originally shared with the DAF on September 21, 2021. The draft report, dated September 2021, was reviewed by formal peer reviewers and DAF subject-matter experts.

Acknowledgments

We are grateful to Col Rudolph Cachuela, Pacific Air Forces (PACAF) Surgeon General, for his guidance and support. We also thank members of his staff, Colonel Mike Foutch, Colonel Jennifer Bein, and James Sandvig, for their ongoing support for this project. We also appreciate the informative context-setting discussions with Col James Sampson at the Air Force Medical Readiness Agency. We especially appreciate the candid engagement on current readiness activities for medical personnel from representatives of the Air Force Surgeon General, as well as Air Force Special Operations Command's Special Operations Surgical Teams; the Center for the Sustainment of Trauma and Readiness Skills, Baltimore; the PACAF Critical Care Air Transport Team; the Sustained Medical and Readiness Trained program; and the U.S. Air Force School of Aerospace Medicine. We also appreciate our RAND teammates—Barbara Bicksler, Bradley DeBlois, and Nelson Lim—who provided counsel, reviewed our work, and assisted with effectively communicating results. Finally, the research team would like to thank Col Mark Ervin, U.S. Air Force (Ret.), and Brad Deblois of RAND for their thoughtful reviews of this report; their feedback improved it immensely.

Summary

Issue

Most U.S. Air Force medical personnel spend their time at military treatment facilities (MTFs) caring for patients whose ailments are far less complex or urgent than the severe trauma-related injuries they would see in war. This mismatch between peacetime and wartime medical care necessitates a deliberate effort on the part of the Air Force Medical Service (AFMS) as a whole, and Pacific Air Forces (PACAF), to ensure that personnel in critical medical specialties receive the training and hands-on clinical experience they need to save lives in a high-casualty environment. The goal of this research project was to investigate approaches for increasing readiness and proficiency.

Approach

To develop a portfolio of readiness building activities, the project team

1. analyzed manpower and personnel data
2. reviewed Comprehensive Medical Readiness Program (CMRP) checklists
3. reviewed relevant literature
4. engaged in discussions with the stakeholder community
5. developed models of the assignment system and of skill acquisition and decay.

In addition, the team developed a prototype framework to demonstrate a possible method for deciding which readiness building activities and assignment policies to employ.

Key Findings

In regard to maintaining clinical proficiency and measuring readiness, we found the following:

- Although personnel assigned to the Western Pacific (WestPac) tend to be more experienced, on average, than those in locations in the continental United States, undermanning combined with skill decay in remote regions can have a significant impact on readiness.
- Deployments have been opportunities to develop proficiency, but these opportunities are declining. The impact on proficiency needs to be better understood, and other options to develop currency and readiness need to be utilized.
- CMRP checklists do not fully function as intended, in part because the requirements are not complete and not consistently defined for all specialties. As a result, there is no real standard against which to measure readiness, measure improvements in knowledge or skills, or identify areas of concern.

In regard to developing a portfolio of readiness building activities, we found the following:

- We could identify no single organization with visibility over the types of readiness activities currently being used throughout the MTFs and major commands, lessons learned, or investments being made and required. As a result, it appears that sharing information on effective readiness initiatives occurs primarily on an ad hoc basis.
- Training activities are perhaps the easiest options to increase currency because they can be focused directly on trauma and critical care, have low manpower costs and time commitment, and require little coordination outside the Air Force.
- Readiness activities in the practice category include a wide variety of options for placing medical personnel in settings that require more-intensive patient care than the typical MTF. The different characteristics of these options accommodate the requirements of different Air Force Specialty Codes (AFSCs) and specialties.
- Assignment policies could contribute to readiness for WestPac without having a negative effect on other locations. Shortening tours, assignment sequencing, and using nonmilitary personnel at low-volume locations produced a meaningful increase in proficiency for several AFSCs.
- Using a systematic framework to match different types of personnel according to their priority ranking, constraints on participation, and constraints on the activities could enable the AFMS to take a holistic view of different strategies for building readiness and how to employ them for different types of personnel.

Recommendations

1. The Air Force should treat the readiness of medical personnel as an enterprise problem requiring an enterprise solution. To implement this recommendation, the AFMS needs to
   a. ensure an organizational entity has the authority and resources to maintain an enterprise-wide view of the proficiency and readiness of medical personnel
   b. develop consistent metrics for reviewing readiness levels across critical medical AFSCs that can be used to monitor personnel in different types of assignments
   c. take a portfolio approach to employing and developing readiness building activities.
2. The AFMS, in collaboration with the Air Force Personnel Center, should view assignments over the course of a career as a key component in the development of the proficiency and readiness of its personnel.
3. PACAF should continue to advocate for activities and policies that enhance proficiency of wartime skills and readiness for potential conflict.
4. The AFMS should undertake a comprehensive assessment of the requirements for medical simulation across the spectrum of modes, levels of complexity, and needed outcomes to include infrastructure and support.

Contents

About This Report iii
Summary v
Figures and Tables viii
Chapter 1. Medical Readiness in a Priority Theater 1
  Loss of Trauma-Related Skills in Peacetime 2
  Research Objective and Approach 5
  The Organization of This Report 7
Chapter 2. Personnel and Readiness Requirements in Critical Medical Specialties 8
  Critical Medical Specialties 8
  Characteristics of Critical Medical Specialties 11
  Readiness Requirements 20
Chapter 3. Readiness Building: Training and Practice Activities 26
  Training Activities 27
  Practice Activities 33
  Chapter Summary 43
Chapter 4. Readiness Building: Assignment Policies 46
  Assignment Policies 46
  Simulating Assignment Policies 48
  The Impact of Assignment Policies 53
  Chapter Summary 60
Chapter 5. A Framework for Matching Personnel to Readiness Activities 61
  Scoring Personnel 61
  Rating Readiness Building Activities 63
  Matching Personnel to Readiness Activities 65
  Chapter Summary 67
Chapter 6. Findings and Recommendations 68
  Findings 68
  Recommendations 69
Appendix A. Assignment Policy Modeling and Simulation Details 72
Appendix B. Reported Cost of Simulation Options 80
Appendix C. A Logic Model for Air Force Medical Service Medical Personnel Currency and Readiness 82
Abbreviations 87
Bibliography 89

Figures and Tables

Figures

Figure 1.1. Research Approach 6
Figure 2.1. The Population of Air Force Medical Personnel 12
Figure 2.2. Average Number of Personnel by Air Force Specialty Code, 2018–2020 13
Figure 2.3. Average Manning Levels by Air Force Specialty Code and Location, 2018–2020 14
Figure 2.4. Average Experience Levels by Air Force Specialty Code and Location, 2018–2020 15
Figure 2.5. Seniority of Officers by Location, 2018–2020 16
Figure 2.6. Seniority of Enlisted Personnel by Location, 2018–2020 17
Figure 2.7. Enlisted Skill Level by Air Force Specialty Code and Location, 2018–2020 18
Figure 2.8. Deployment Rates by Air Force Specialty Code, 2018–2020 19
Figure 4.1. The Modeling and Simulation Methodology 49
Figure 4.2. Simulated Proficiency for Two Individuals over 96 Months 52
Figure 4.3. Average Proficiency by Location Category 57
Figure 4.4. Average Proficiency of Individuals in the Western Pacific, by Air Force Specialty Code and Simulation 59
Figure 5.1. Algorithm for Matching Types of Personnel to Readiness Activities 65
Figure A.1. Assignment Flows into the Western Pacific for Career Field 4N0X1 73
Figure A.2. Cumulative Probability That an Individual Is Retained in an Existing Assignment over Time, by Western Pacific Location 74
Figure A.3. Cumulative Continuation Rates for Career Field 4N0X1 74
Figure A.4. Average Proficiency of Individuals in the Western Pacific by Air Force Specialty Code and Simulation for Model with High Learning Rate and Low Decay Rate 76
Figure A.5. Average Proficiency of Individuals in the Western Pacific by Air Force Specialty Code and Simulation for Model with High Learning Rate and High Decay Rate 77
Figure A.6. Average Proficiency of Individuals in the Western Pacific by Air Force Specialty Code and Simulation for Model with Low Learning Rate and Low Decay Rate 78
Figure A.7. Average Proficiency of Individuals in the Western Pacific by Air Force Specialty Code and Simulation for Model with Low Learning Rate and High Decay Rate 79
Figure C.1. The Logic Model for Air Force Medical Service Personnel Currency and Readiness 84

Tables

Table 2.1. Air Force Critical Medical Career Fields Included in This Study ... 9
Table 2.2. Air Force Critical Medical Career Fields Shredouts ... 10
Table 3.1. Readiness Building Activities and Policies ... 27
Table 3.2. Characteristics of Training and Practice Readiness Building Activities ... 44
Table 4.1. Percentage of Assignments Originating from Tier 1 Locations ... 55
Table 5.1. The Scheme for Prioritizing Personnel ... 62
Table 5.2. The Scheme for Rating Readiness Building Activities ... 63
Table A.1. Regional and Proficiency Tier Classifications by Base and Location ... 72
Table B.1. Reported Costs of Simulation Options ... 80

Chapter 1. Medical Readiness in a Priority Theater

The Pacific region is a priority theater for both the U.S. Air Force and the U.S. military as a whole. The region features multiple security challenges, and Pacific Air Forces (PACAF) seek to be ready to "fight tonight" if the need arises.[1] The U.S. Air Force Strategic Master Plan identifies the Pacific as a "region of increased national emphasis."[2] Similarly, the head of the U.S. Indo-Pacific Command recently testified to Congress that the Pacific is "the most consequential region for America's future . . . [it] remains the DoD's priority theater . . . [and it] contains four of the five priority security challenges identified by DoD."[3] The U.S. Department of Defense (DoD) has increasingly emphasized that the effort to counter China is its top military priority.[4]

If conflict were to break out in the Pacific, Air Force medical personnel would be called upon to care for a broad range of trauma injuries in a potentially contested environment with limited resources.[5] Providing immediate and effective care for the injured would often mean the difference between life or death. This fact was made clear during U.S. military operations in Afghanistan and Iraq, in which nearly 1,000 U.S. military personnel died of "potentially survivable" injuries between 2001 and 2011. Nearly all (91 percent) of these deaths were associated with hemorrhage, with most of the remaining deaths associated with airway obstruction (8 percent).[6] Fatality rates were highest early on, with trauma care capabilities improving throughout the course of these conflicts.[7] In addition to preventing fatalities, optimal combat casualty care is needed to prevent

[1] PACAF, "Info," webpage, undated.

[2] U.S. Air Force, *USAF Strategic Master Plan*, May 2015.

[3] Philip S. Davidson, "U.S. Indo-Pacific Command Posture," statement before the Committee on Armed Services, U.S. Senate, March 9, 2021.

[4] Jacqueline Feldscher, "China Is Our No. 1 Priority. Start Acting Like It, Austin Tells Pentagon," *Defense One*, June 9, 2021; Reuters, "Remember: 'China, China, China,' New Acting U.S. Defense Secretary Says," January 2, 2019; Ronald O'Rourke, *Renewed Great Power Competition: Implications for Defense—Issues for Congress*, Congressional Research Service, R43838, August 3, 2021, p. 3; DoD, *Summary of the 2018 National Defense Strategy of the United States of America: Sharpening the American Military's Competitive Edge*, 2018.

[5] Brent Thomas, *Preparing for the Future of Combat Casualty Care: Opportunities to Refine the Military Health System's Alignment with the National Defense Strategy*, RAND Corporation, RR-A713-1, 2021.

[6] Brian J. Eastridge, Robert L. Mabry, Peter Seguin, Joyce Cantrell, Terrill Tops, Paul Uribe, Olga Mallett, Tamara Zubko, Lynne Oetjen-Gerdes, Todd E. Rasmussen, Frank K Butler, Russell S. Kotwal, John B. Holcomb, Charles Wade, Howard Champion, Mimi Lawnick, Leon Moores, and Lorne H. Blackbourne, "Death on the Battlefield (2001–2011): Implications for the Future of Combat Casualty Care," *Journal of Trauma and Acute Care Surgery*, Vol. 73, No. 6, December 2012, pp. S431, S434–S435.

[7] Donald Berwick, Autumn Downey, and Elizabeth Cornett, eds., *A National Trauma Care System: Integrating Military and Civilian Trauma Systems to Achieve Zero Preventable Deaths After Injury*, National Academies Press, 2016, pp. 50–53.

deterioration and facilitate recovery from battlefield injuries such as spinal cord injury, traumatic brain injury, and vascular injuries to limbs.[8]

As suggested by the PACAF Surgeon General, this report focuses on critical medical specialties needed to treat wartime trauma, including emergency physicians, surgeons, anesthesiologists, physician assistants, nurses, surgical services, and medical technicians. Active-duty personnel assigned to PACAF in these critical medical specialties bear primary responsibility for caring for wounded airmen.[9] This includes 639 active-duty medical personnel stationed in Guam, Japan, and South Korea, in locations that could be among the first to see casualties in the event of conflict. Another 554 medical personnel are stationed in Alaska or Hawaii, where they are available to quickly deploy to provide frontline medical support or to provide on-site care for casualties evacuated to the United States. Together, these 1,193 critical medical personnel assigned to PACAF represent 11.6 percent of the 10,325 critical medical personnel on active duty in the Air Force as a whole.

Loss of Trauma-Related Skills in Peacetime

With the end of major military operations in Afghanistan and Iraq, fewer and fewer Air Force Medical Service (AFMS) personnel have experience providing wartime care. Most AFMS personnel are assigned to in-garrison medical treatment facilities (MTFs) in the United States. Ideally, the care they provide to service members, dependents, and other beneficiaries would enable AFMS personnel to maintain skills necessary for wartime readiness. However, most MTF care consists of providing routine, preventive, and outpatient services with little resemblance to wartime care. Even in MTF inpatient facilities, the most common procedures are related to pregnancy, childbirth, and newborn care.[10] While practicing at MTFs, military medical personnel very rarely perform trauma care procedures such as hemorrhage management, resuscitation, and wound debridement.[11]

---

[8] Kevin F. Fitzpatrick and Paul F. Pasquina, "Overview of the Rehabilitation of the Combat Casualty," *Military Medicine*, Vol. 175, No. 7S, July 2010; Michael S. Jaffee, Kathy M. Helmick, Philip D. Girard, Kim S. Meyer, Kathy Dinegar, and Karyn George, "Acute Clinical Care and Care Coordination for Traumatic Brain Injury within Department of Defense," *Journal of Rehabilitation Research and Development*, Vol. 46, No. 6, 2009; Yichi Xu, Wenjing Xu, Aiyuan Wang, Haoye Meng, Yu Wang, Shuyun Liu, Rui Li, Shibi Lu, and Jiang Peng, "Diagnosis and Treatment of Traumatic Vascular Injury of Limbs in Military and Emergency Medicine: A Systematic Review," *Medicine*, Vol. 98, No. 18, May 2019.

[9] We identified 14 Air Force Specialty Codes (AFSCs) that are critical to providing combat care (for details, see Chapter 2). Counts are based on the number of individuals assigned to positions in these critical medical specialties at the start of fiscal year (FY) 2021.

[10] Berwick, Downey, and Cornett, 2016, pp. 243–244.

[11] Edward W. Chan, Heather Krull, Sangeeta C. Ahluwalia, James R. Broyles, Daniel A. Waxman, Jill Gurvey, Paul M. Colthirst, JoEllen Schimmels, and Anthony Marinos, *Options for Maintaining Clinical Proficiency During Peacetime*, RAND Corporation, RR-2543-A, 2020, pp. 23–24.

Given this mismatch between peacetime care and wartime care, the Air Force and other military services have long struggled to ensure that medical personnel have the training and experience necessary to care effectively for service members injured in combat. Though all Air Force personnel in critical medical specialties go through an initial training period, the skills they learn relevant to trauma care fade over time if not regularly practiced.

Skill decay is defined as the loss of skills or knowledge after periods of nonuse that affects a broad array of tasks, and it includes a loss of the declarative knowledge (knowing *what*—i.e., knowledge about facts) and procedural knowledge (knowing *how*) that constitute critical medical skills.[12] Multiple factors influence the rate of skill decay, including the period of skill nonuse, the degree of overlearning involved in acquiring the skill (i.e., training beyond that required for initial currency), task characteristics, methods of testing for initial learning and retention, conditions of retrieval, instructional strategies and training methods, and individual differences in learners.[13]

The military has long observed and measured skill decay across professions; in a general example that was not specific to medical professionals, a study of 20,000 reservists revealed that gross motor skills decayed after ten months, and cognitive skills decayed within about six months.[14] Recent skill decay literature documents the effect of skill decay on medical skills ranging from basic skills like cardiopulmonary resuscitation (CPR) to more complex skills like advanced cardiac life support, diagnostic skills, and surgical tasks. Among laypeople, CPR skills begin to deteriorate "within weeks to months of certification and continue to decline over time"; among paramedics and emergency medical technicians, these types of skills decrease after certification, as do more complex skills, such as endotracheal tube insertions.[15] Among nurses, emergency resuscitation skills decline as soon as ten weeks after training;[16] nurses in one study had a 14-percent pass rate for advanced cardiac life support at the 12-month reassessment mark.[17]

---

[12] Winfred Arthur, Jr., Winston Bennett, Jr., Pamela L. Stanush, and Theresa L. McNelly, "Factors That Influence Skill Decay and Retention: A Quantitative Review and Analysis," *Human Performance*, Vol. 11, No. 1, 1998.

[13] Ray S. Perez, Anna Skinner, Peter Weyhrauch, James Niehaus, Corinna Lathan, Steven D. Schwaitzberg, and Caroline G. L. Cao, "Prevention of Surgical Skill Decay," *Military Medicine*, Vol. 178, No. 10S, October 2013.

[14] Robert Wisher, Mark Sabol, and John Ellis, *Staying Sharp: Retention of Military Knowledge and Skills*, U.S. Army Research Institute Special Report 39, July 1999.

[15] Alexandra L. Rhue and Beth VanDerveer, "Wilderness First Responder: Are Skills Soon Forgotten?" *Wilderness and Environmental Medicine*, Vol. 29, No. 1, March 2018.

[16] Rebecca Broomfield, "A Quasi-Experimental Research to Investigate the Retention of Basic Cardiopulmonary Resuscitation Skills and Knowledge by Qualified Nurses Following a Course in Professional Development," *Journal of Advanced Nursing*, Vol. 23, No. 5, June 28, 2008; Catherine Madden, "Undergraduate Nursing Students' Acquisition and Retention of CPR Knowledge and Skills," *Nurse Education Today*, Vol. 26, No. 3, April 2006.

[17] Kimberly K. Smith, Darlene Gilcreast, and Karen Pierce, "Evaluation of Staff's Retention of ACLS and BLS Skills," *Resuscitation*, Vol. 78, No. 1, July 2008.

Nurses and other health professionals trained in newborn life support have decreased skills as early as three to five months after training.[18]

Skill decay in medicine applies broadly; according to one study, "practicing physicians and residents tended to mirror the skill and knowledge retention declines found in medical students, lay individuals, and other health care providers."[19] Skill in paracentesis, a method for removing fluid from the body cavity, declines as early as three months after training,[20] and skill at obtaining a transthoracic echocardiogram—a noninvasive but complex procedure—among participants in one study decayed after only 11 days.[21] Skill decay also contributes to diagnostic error, defined as cases where diagnoses were inaccurate, unintentionally delayed, or absent.[22]

Erosion during peacetime of medical skills needed to treat the kinds of casualties received during a war is a particular problem that one set of authors called the "Peacetime Effect":

> Once fighting ends, wartime surgeons and medical specialists disperse, casualty care systems dismantle, military specific publications in the medical literature significantly decline, and the focus on injury-related education and training wanes. During these times, Military Health System (MHS) leaders prioritize the mission of wellness among active duty members and other beneficiaries over combat-relevant training. Then, when the military mobilizes for the next war, the MHS is ill equipped for combat and its members are unprepared to manage casualties.[23]

As the literature on skill decay suggests, military medical personnel practicing at MTFs are likely to experience decay of the knowledge and skills that they will need to save lives during emergency situations.[24] Without appropriate battlefield readiness among Air Force medical personnel, service members are at risk for experiencing unnecessary morbidity and mortality during wartime. Yet this reality is unsurprising. One should not assume that providing peacetime

---

[18] C. M. J. Mosley and B. N. J. Shaw, "A Longitudinal Cohort Study to Investigate the Retention of Knowledge and Skills Following Attendance on the Newborn Life Support Course," *Archives of Disease in Childhood*, Vol. 98, No. 8, August 1, 2013.

[19] Rhue and VanDerveer, 2018.

[20] Dana Sall, Eric J. Warm, Benjamin Kinnear, Matthew Kelleher, Roman Jandarov, and Jennifer O'Toole, "See One, Do One, Forget One: Early Skill Decay After Paracentesis Training," *Journal of General Internal Medicine*, Vol. 36, No. 5, May 2021.

[21] Dario Cecilio-Fernandes, Fokie Cnossen, Debbie A. D. C. Jaarsma, and René A. Tio, "Avoiding Surgical Skill Decay: A Systematic Review on the Spacing of Training Sessions," *Journal of Surgical Education*, Vol. 75, No. 2, March 2018.

[22] Sallie J. Weaver, David E. Newman-Toker, and Michael A. Rosen, "Reducing Cognitive Skill Decay and Diagnostic Error: Theory-Based Practices for Continuing Education in Health Care," *Journal of Continuing Education in the Health Professions*, Vol. 32, No. 4, 2012.

[23] Jeremy W. Cannon, Kirby R. Gross, and Todd E. Rasmussen, "Combating the Peacetime Effect in Military Medicine," *JAMA Surgery*, September 2020, p. E1.

[24] Brandon M. Carius, Michael D. April, and Steve G. Schauer, "Procedural Volume Within Military Treatment Facilities—Implications for a Ready Medical Force," *Military Medicine*, Vol. 185, Nos. 7–8, July–August 2020.

health care in an MTF is sufficient to ensure wartime readiness any more than one would assume that flying for passenger airlines is sufficient to ensure a trained fighter pilot.

Rather, medical personnel will need to participate in additional activities to ensure readiness. To the extent that this detracts from the provision of peacetime health care or requires additional investment, it should be seen as the cost of ensuring readiness. The AFMS and certain major commands (MAJCOMs) and MTFs have introduced programs and initiatives to provide additional training and practice for trauma and critical care skills (some of which are described in Chapter 3); however, these may not be sufficient and have been organized and resourced on an ad hoc basis.

Reforms have been underway since the establishment of the Defense Health Agency (DHA) in 2013, with the goal of these reforms being to consolidate medical administration, training, and logistics in the medical commands of the armed services. In 2017, the U.S. Congress gave the DHA broad authority for facilities and for the provision of medical care to family members and retirees. As of March 2022, the DHA has plans for major changes to many military health facilities. For example, 37 will no longer see civilian patients.[25] Further adjustments by the DHA will also affect the ability of the services to maintain the readiness of medical personnel.

Senior AFMS leadership must accept and program for the cost of ensuring readiness and ensure subordinate commands demonstrate that wartime readiness is the driving principle for medical readiness. In addition, many of the actions called for in this report will be beyond the ability of PACAF and the AFMS to carry out on their own. Coordination with the U.S. Air Force as a whole and the DHA will be required.

Research Objective and Approach

PACAF is not always assigned individuals in critical medical specialties who have the skills needed to provide effective care in both peacetime and wartime, and it faces challenges in ensuring that these individuals are able to maintain their skills over time. The readiness of medical personnel to provide effective care for the injured in the PACAF area of responsibility depends on the readiness of personnel assigned to PACAF in peacetime and those who deploy to PACAF in time of conflict. From PACAF's perspective, these personnel need high levels of proficiency and readiness. Therefore, RAND Project AIR FORCE was asked to examine these challenges and to investigate approaches for increasing and maintaining readiness for critical medical specialties across the entire AFMS.

Figure 1.1 depicts the steps the research team took in conducting our analysis. We began by analyzing manpower and personnel data to better understand the characteristics of medical professionals in critical medical specialties and the authorized manpower positions in which they

[25] Patricia Kime, "Plans for Hospital Closures as Part of Military Health System Reform Forging Ahead After Pause," Military.com, March 30, 2022.

serve. Next, we reviewed Comprehensive Medical Readiness Program (CMRP) checklists in order to compare the consistency and adequacy of readiness requirements across AFSCs.

Figure 1.1. Research Approach

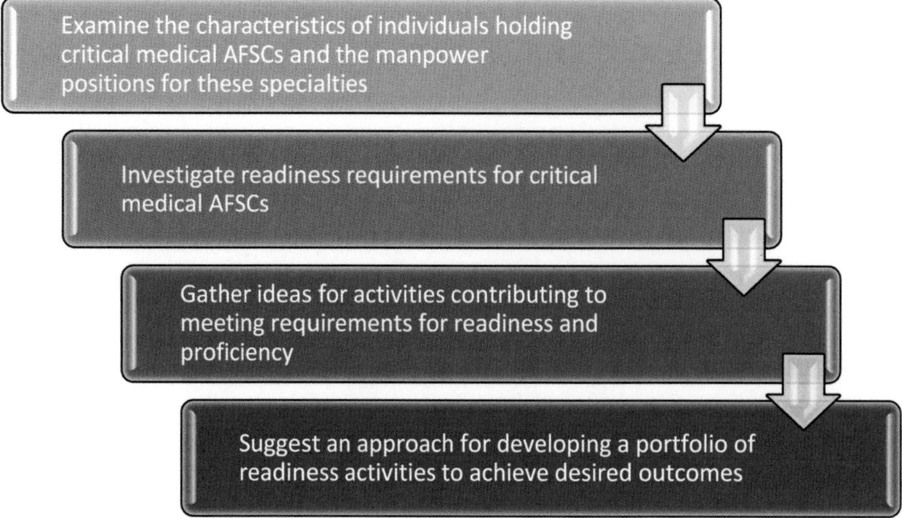

Third, by reviewing relevant literature and engaging in discussions with representatives from Air Force medical organizations, the team gathered a list of potential activities that could be implemented to increase the readiness and proficiency of individuals in critical medical specialties. We arranged these activities into three categories:

1. *Training activities:* didactic education that may or may not include hands-on experience, such as precepted (instructor-supervised) patient care or simulated patient care.
2. *Practice activities:* opportunities to provide nonprecepted, direct patient care for trauma and critical care patients with the intent of improving wartime medical knowledge and performance of key procedures.
3. *Assignment policies*: options for tailoring the order, length, or location of a medical provider's assignments to help maintain wartime knowledge and performance.

Training and practice activities would be undertaken in addition to or instead of their assignments to in-garrison MTFs. We developed a comprehensive list of such activities and investigated each to describe the characteristics. To assess the effect of assignment initiatives on proficiency, the research team developed a simulation model of the assignment system combined with a computational cognitive model of skill acquisition and decay.

Finally, the team developed and demonstrated an approach that can be used by the AFMS to systematically determine which activities to consider establishing or expanding and then resourcing. Using this approach, we illustrate how to prioritize specific groups of medical personnel and match them to readiness building activities.

The Organization of This Report

The remainder of this report contains the results of our research. Chapter 2 provides an overview and demographics for critical medical AFSCs and reviews the Air Force's medical readiness requirements for each AFSC. In Chapter 3 we introduce a set of readiness building activities and policies and, for those activities related to training and practice, describe the activity and how it would boost readiness for medical personnel. Chapter 4 turns to assignment policies and reports on how these readiness building policies contribute to proficiency. Chapter 5 describes a systematic approach to assigning readiness building activities to medical personnel and employs this approach using the Western Pacific (WestPac) as an example. We conclude, in Chapter 6, with recommendations.

Chapter 2. Personnel and Readiness Requirements in Critical Medical Specialties

The AFMS is made up of approximately 20,000 active-duty enlisted personnel and 7,000 officers.[1] These individuals are assigned to more than 80 medical career fields that contain dozens of specialties.[2] The requisite knowledge, skills, and abilities (KSAs) vary widely across AFMS career fields and range from providing comprehensive medical care to service members and family units, to providing specialized surgical services, to managing and assisting with all facets of medical care.[3]

The educational and training requirements also vary widely from completion of high school or General Education Development equivalency, to completion of a bachelor's or master's degree from an accredited program, to completion of a doctor of medicine degree along with residencies, fellowships, and board certifications. The great diversity of skills across medical career fields and specialties is necessary for the AFMS to meet the mission of ensuring medically fit forces, providing expeditionary medics, and serving beneficiary populations.

This chapter describes the current state of active-duty medical personnel along with the set of activities they must perform to build and sustain clinical currency and readiness. We begin by defining the subset of critical medical AFSCs. We then compare authorizations, end strength, and experience by AFSC and location. Finally, we review readiness requirements by AFSC as expressed in CMRP checklists, the system used to ensure readiness to provide care in wartime.

Critical Medical Specialties

Our analysis of medical personnel readiness did not include all medical AFSCs. Instead, we worked with the project sponsor to identify a *subset of critical medical AFSCs* on which to focus. Some of these AFSCs have a low number of funded authorizations (i.e., a low density) that nevertheless provide services that would be in high demand in the event of conflict.[4] Other included AFSCs are considered critical operational specialties and are, for example, given priority for trauma training. Table 2.1 lists the 14 critical medical career fields that were the

---

[1] Values are based on officer and enlisted personnel extracts taken from the Military Personnel Data System at the start of FY 2021.

[2] Air Force Personnel Center (AFPC), *Air Force Enlisted Classification Directory (AFECD): The Official Guide to the Air Force Enlisted Classification Codes*, April 30, 2021a; AFPC, *Air Force Officer Classification Directory (AFOCD): The Official Guide to the Air Force Officer Classification Codes*, April 30, 2021b.

[3] AFPC, 2021a; AFPC, 2021b.

[4] We did not analyze unit type codes (UTCs) slated for WestPac operations plans. Any requirements for medical personnel in WestPac should consider these operations plans.

focus of the study. We further divided three career fields (46NX, 46YX, and 4N0X1) into trauma and critical care providers and nontrauma and noncritical care providers based on specialties (referred to as shredouts within the AFSCs), bringing the total number of career field groupings to 17 (see Table 2.2).

Table 2.1. Air Force Critical Medical Career Fields Included in This Study

AFSC	Title	Specialty Description
Officer AFSCs		
42GX	Physician Assistant	Provides comprehensive health maintenance and continuing medical care to assigned patient population. Examines, diagnoses, and treats diseases and injuries.
44EX	Emergency Services Physician	Examines, diagnoses, and treats initial and acute phase of illnesses and injuries. Directs emergency and related outpatient services. Directs disaster planning, training, and management in the prehospital and hospital access areas.
44FX	Family Physician	Provides continuing, comprehensive health maintenance and medical care to entire family. Directs outpatient and inpatient care and services. Instructs other health care providers and nonmedical personnel.
44MX	Internist	Diagnoses diseases and renders nonsurgical care; provides consultation in complex cases.
45AX	Anesthesiologist	Administers general and local anesthetics; manages anesthesiology services.
45BX	Orthopedic Surgeon	Examines, diagnoses, and treats diseases and injuries of musculoskeletal system by surgical and conservative means.
45SX	Surgeon	Examines, diagnoses, and treats, by surgical and conservative means, diseases, and injuries.
46NX	Clinical Nurse	Provides professional nursing care. Acts as patient advocate and advances desired health outcomes through patient and family education.
46SX	Operating Room Nurse	Assesses, plans, implements, and evaluates perioperative nursing care. Plans, directs, and coordinates activities of the Operating Room Department.
46YX	Advanced Practice Registered Nurse	Provides professional nursing care. Acts as patient advocate and advances desired health outcomes through patient/family education.
48RX	Residency Trained Flight Surgeon	Administers the aerospace medicine program; conducts medical examinations and provides medical care for aircrews, missile crews, special duty operators, and others with special standards of medical qualification and readiness functions. Evaluates living and working environments to control health hazards and prevent disease and injury.
Enlisted AFSCs		
4H0X1	Cardiopulmonary Laboratory	Performs and manages cardiopulmonary laboratory functions and activities for respiratory care services, noninvasive diagnostic cardiac procedures, invasive diagnostic and interventional cardiac procedures, pulmonary function testing, and diagnostic and therapeutic bronchoscopies.
4N0X1	Aerospace Medical Service	Plans, provides, and evaluates routine patient care and treatment of beneficiaries, to include flying and special operational duty personnel.
4N1X1	Surgical Service	Participates in and manages the planning, provision, and evaluation of surgical patient care activities and related training programs.

SOURCES: AFPC, 2021a; AFPC, 2021b.
NOTE: The *X* in the AFSC can be filled by a digit to indicate the level of qualification of the individual holding the AFSC (e.g., entry, qualified, member for officers and helper, apprentice, journeyman, craftsman, superintendent for enlisted members).

Table 2.2. Air Force Critical Medical Career Fields Shredouts

Officer AFSCs

42GX Physician Assistant
- A – Orthopedics
- B – Otolaryngology
- C – General Surgery
- E – Emergency Medicine
- N – Psychiatry
- P – Aerospace Operational Medicine

44EX Emergency Services Physician
- A – Emergency Medicine Specialist

44FX Family Physician
- A – Sports Medicine
- B – Obstetrics
- C – Pain Management

44MX Internist
- A – Oncology
- B – Cardiology
- C – Endocrinology
- D – Gastroenterology
- E – Hematology
- F – Rheumatology
- G – Pulmonary Diseases
- H – Infectious Diseases
- J – Nephrology
- K – Geriatrics/Palliative Care Medicine
- L – Sleep Medicine

45AX Anesthesiologist
- A – Cardiothoracic
- B – Pain Management

45BX Orthopedic Surgeon
- A – Hand Surgery
- B – Pediatrics
- D – Sports Medicine
- E – Spine Surgery
- F – Oncology
- G – Replacement Arthroplasty
- H – Traumatology

45SX Surgeon
- A – Thoracic
- B – Colon and Rectal
- C – Cardiac
- D – Pediatric
- E – Peripheral Vascular
- F – Neurological
- G – Plastic
- H – Oncology
- K – Trauma/Critical Care

46NX Clinical Nurse

Trauma and critical care
- E – Critical Care
- J – Emergency/Trauma

Nontrauma and critical care
- D – Staff Development
- F – Neonatal Intensive Care
- G – Obstetrical

46SX Operating Room Nurse

None

46YX Advanced Practice Registered Nurse

Trauma and critical care
- C – Acute Care Nurse Practitioner
- M – Certified Registered Nurse Anesthetist

Nontrauma and critical care
- A – Women's Health Care Nurse Practitioner
- B – Pediatric Nurse Practitioner
- F – Aeromedical Nurse Practitioner
- G – Certified Nurse Midwife
- H – Family Nurse Practitioner
- P – Adult Psychiatric and Mental Health Nurse

48RX Residency-Trained Flight Surgeon
- E – Board eligible in emergency medicine
- F – Board eligible in family medicine
- M – Board eligible in internal medicine

Enlisted AFSCs

4H0X1 Cardiopulmonary Laboratory

None

4N0X1 Aerospace Medical Service

Trauma and critical care
- C – Independent Duty Medical Technician (IDMT)

Nontrauma and critical care
- B – Neurodiagnostic Medical Technician
- F – Flight and Operational Medical Technician

4N1X1 Surgical Service
- B – Urology
- C – Orthopedics
- D – Otolaryngology

SOURCES: AFPC, 2021a; AFPC, 2021b.

NOTE: Shredouts listed are appended to AFSCs as suffixes if applicable. To highlight trauma and critical care specialties, we divided three career fields (46NX, 46YX, and 4N0X1) into trauma and critical care providers and nontrauma and noncritical care providers. Some practitioners in other subspecialties may require significant clinical exposure outside their chosen subspecialty to maintain clinical proficiency in deployment-related skills.

Individuals in AFMS career fields are assigned to hundreds of Air Force and military locations in the continental United States (CONUS) and outside the continental United States (OCONUS). The services offered by MTFs at these locations vary and, by extension, so do the opportunities they provide medical professionals to build and sustain clinical proficiency. The AFMS has approximately 80 MTFs, which are part of the more than 50 full-service hospitals and 370 clinics that make up the MHS. Broadly, these facilities are divided among three types—medical centers, hospitals, and clinics.[5]

Medical centers are the largest type of military MTF. Medical centers offer hospitalization and outpatient services, house multiple specialties and subspecialties, may serve as trauma centers (in a few cases offering Level 1 or Level 2 trauma care), and may participate in general medical education and medical research programs. Hospitals (or inpatient clinics) are smaller than medical centers. Hospitals offer hospitalization and outpatient services, and they house multiple specialties but not subspecialties. Finally, clinics are the smallest MTFs. They only offer outpatient services, and they house a limited number of specialties.

While the need for medical professionals to maintain readiness to support conflicts with varying amounts of time to prepare varies by location, the time constraints still require deliberate plans to maintain proficiency even in peacetime. At one extreme, personnel assigned to PACAF must stand ready to provide lifesaving care from the onset of unexpected conflict. This requirement is particularly true for individuals assigned to locations in WestPac (i.e., Gaum, Japan, and South Korea). Additionally, individuals stationed in Alaska and Hawaii must be prepared to quickly deploy to provide frontline support or on-site care for medical evacuees. Finally, individuals stationed in CONUS must also be prepared to deploy promptly to support a long-duration or high-intensity conflict.

Characteristics of Critical Medical Specialties

Of the approximately 27,000 active-duty Air Force medical personnel, around 10,000 belong to the critical medical specialties described previously, including 1,193 personnel in critical medical specialties assigned to PACAF, as illustrated in Figure 2.1. In the following sections we examine manning levels, experience levels, and deployment tempo by AFSC and location. For purposes of analysis, we grouped locations into one of four categories based on region: WestPac, Alaska and Hawaii, all other OCONUS, and CONUS.[6]

---

[5] TRICARE, "Types of Military Facilities," webpage, June 15, 2021.

[6] These locations are where individuals are permanently assigned; Air Force members deploy from their home stations. Locations designated "all other OCONUS" are primarily in Europe.

Figure 2.1. The Population of Air Force Medical Personnel

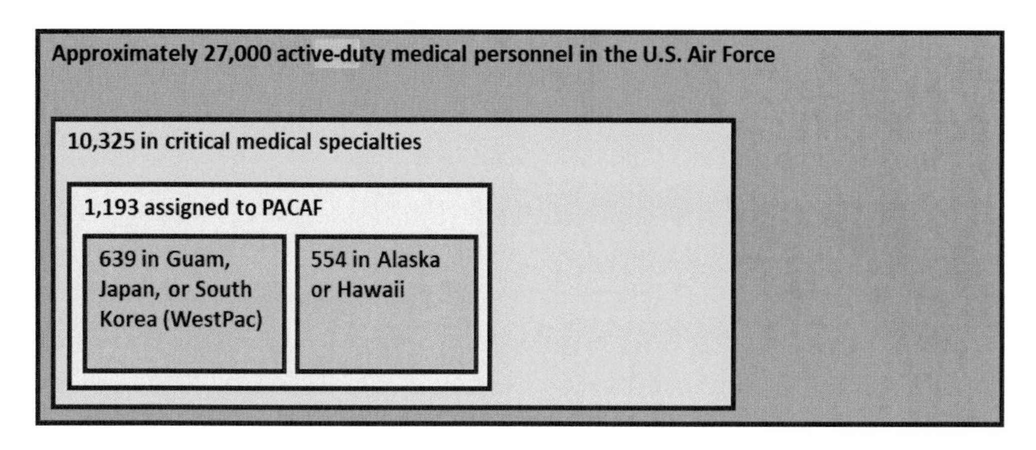

NOTE: Counts are based on the number of individuals assigned to positions in critical medical specialties at the start of FY 2021. Figure is not drawn to scale.

Assignments by Air Force Specialty Code and Location

The average number of individuals assigned to critical medical career fields varies by AFSC and region, as illustrated in Figure 2.2.[7] Of the enlisted AFSCs, Aerospace Medical Service, 4N0X1, contained the most individuals. Of the officer AFSCs, Clinical Nurses, 46NX, contained the most individuals. At the other extreme, surgical specialties (Anesthesiologist, 45AX; Orthopedic Surgeon, 45BX; and Surgeon, 45SX) and Emergency Services Physicians, 44EX contained only dozens of individuals AFMS-wide.

Most individuals are assigned to CONUS locations, which would be expected given the greater number of CONUS military locations and authorizations. Consequently, fewer than five individuals are stationed throughout all of WestPac for certain critical specialties (e.g., three Emergency Services Physicians, 44EX; three Anesthesiologists, 45AX; three Orthopedic Surgeons, 45BX; and three Surgeons, 45SX). This underscores the low number of individuals who are forward assigned with skills that would be in extremely high demand during a conflict.

---

[7] We gathered officer and enlisted personnel extracts from the Military Personnel Data System from the start of each fiscal year for FY 2018–FY 2020. We categorized personnel in this analysis by their duty AFSCs—that is, the AFSCs attached to the positions in which the individuals were serving—since this most closely reflects the kinds of skills needed for the job the individuals currently held. However, we recognize that there may be mismatches between the individuals' primary AFSCs (the specialty that they are best qualified to perform) and their duty AFSCs. Our analysis was exploratory; further analyses should be conducted for a more detailed perspective on the numbers and types of skills in the population.

Figure 2.2. Average Number of Personnel by Air Force Specialty Code, 2018–2020

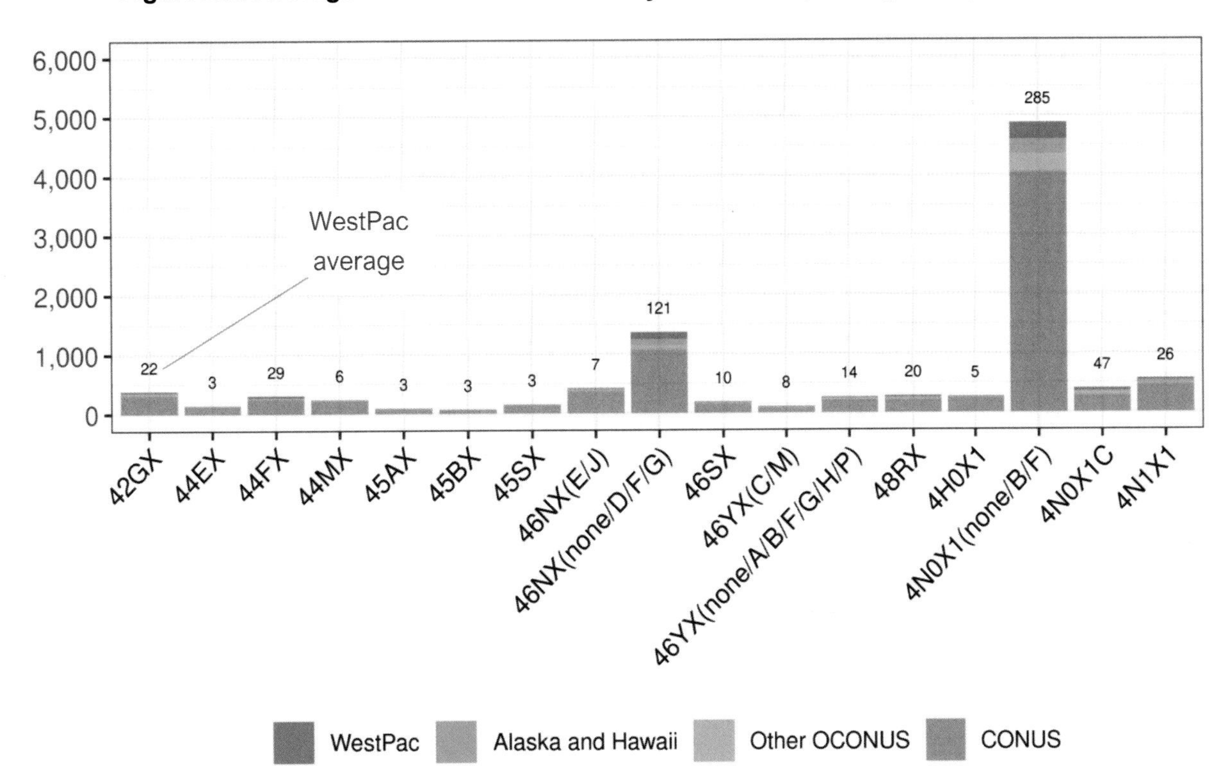

Manning Levels by Air Force Specialty Code and Location

Figure 2.3 shows the manning for critical AFSCs by region. AFSCs with manning levels lower than 80 percent are considered critically undermanned; fully manned AFSCs could have manning levels above 100 percent.[8] Many AFSCs were undermanned, and this varied by location. On average, manning levels were lower at CONUS locations than elsewhere; four AFSCs were critically undermanned, 13 were undermanned, and one was fully manned. In comparison, two AFSCs were critically undermanned in WestPac, six were undermanned, and the remaining nine were fully manned. Manning levels at other OCONUS locations and in Alaska and Hawaii fell in between these values.

[8] These manning thresholds are similar to those used in a recent Government Accountability Office report on military medical personnel manning levels; see Brenda S. Farrell, *Military Personnel: Additional Actions Needed to Address Gaps in Military Physician Specialties*, U.S. Government Accountability Office, GAO-18-77, 2018.

Figure 2.3. Average Manning Levels by Air Force Specialty Code and Location, 2018–2020

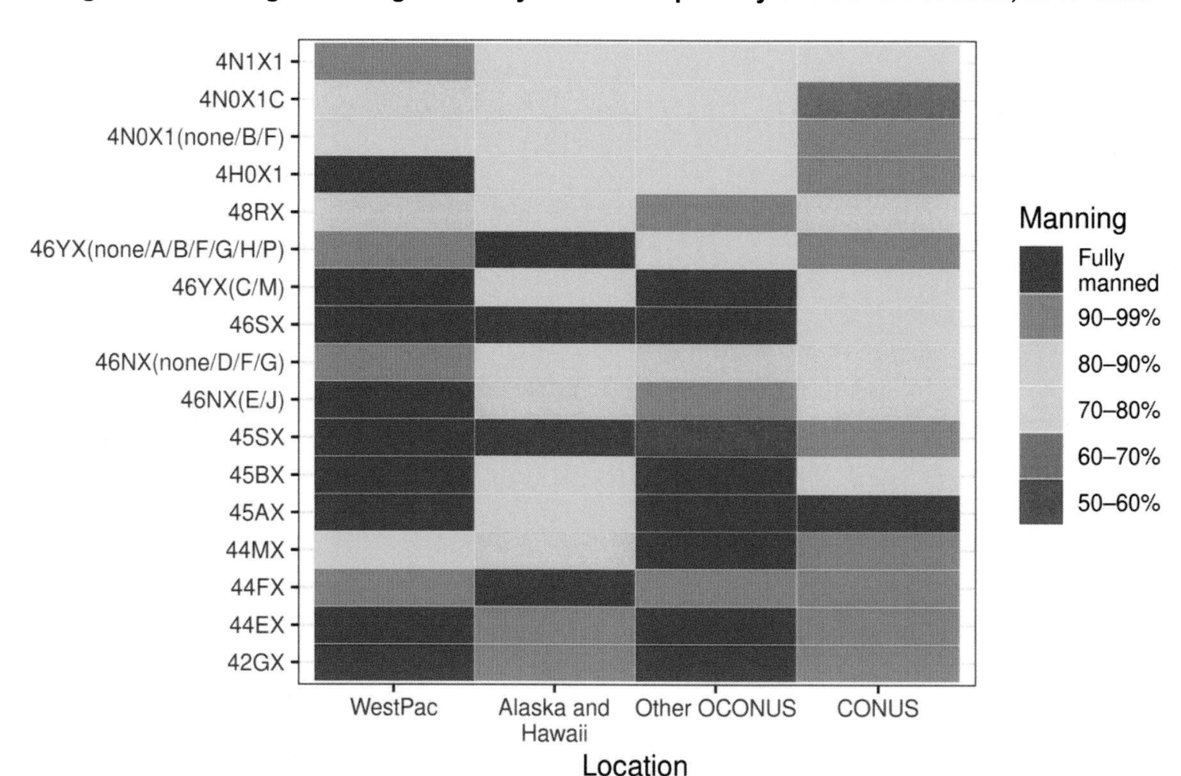

NOTE: In this figure we count as fully manned those AFSCs with an average manning level at or above 100 percent. In five instances, the average number of assigned individuals exceeds authorized positions by exactly one; in two instances there are three more assigned than authorized.

Experience Levels by Air Force Specialty Code and Location

Overall, experience levels, as measured by years of service (YOS), varied by career field and, to a lesser extent, by location, as shown in Figure 2.4. Controlling for differences in location, the specialties with the highest experience levels were Aerospace Medical Service IDMT, 4N0X1(C), followed by Advanced Practice Registered Nurse, 46YX(C/M). Experience levels were lowest for Emergency Services Physician, 44EX, followed by Clinical Nurse, 46NX(E/J).[9] Controlling for differences in career fields, medical personnel assigned to WestPac were somewhat more experienced relative to CONUS locations (the red bars versus the purple bars in Figure 2.4), but

[9] To estimate these values, we performed a logistic regression treating YOS as the outcome and AFSC and location as the predictor variables. The marginal changes in YOS associated with 4N0X1(C) and 46YX(C/M) equaled 4.8 and 4.4 years, respectively; and the marginal changes associated with 44EX and 46NX(E/J) equaled –2.2 and –2.1 years, respectively. In other words, 46YX(C/M) had about 4.4 more years of experience on average, and 44EX had about 2.1 fewer years of experience on average.

less experienced relative to other OCONUS locations (the red bars versus the green bars in Figure 2.4).[10]

Figure 2.4. Average Experience Levels by Air Force Specialty Code and Location, 2018–2020

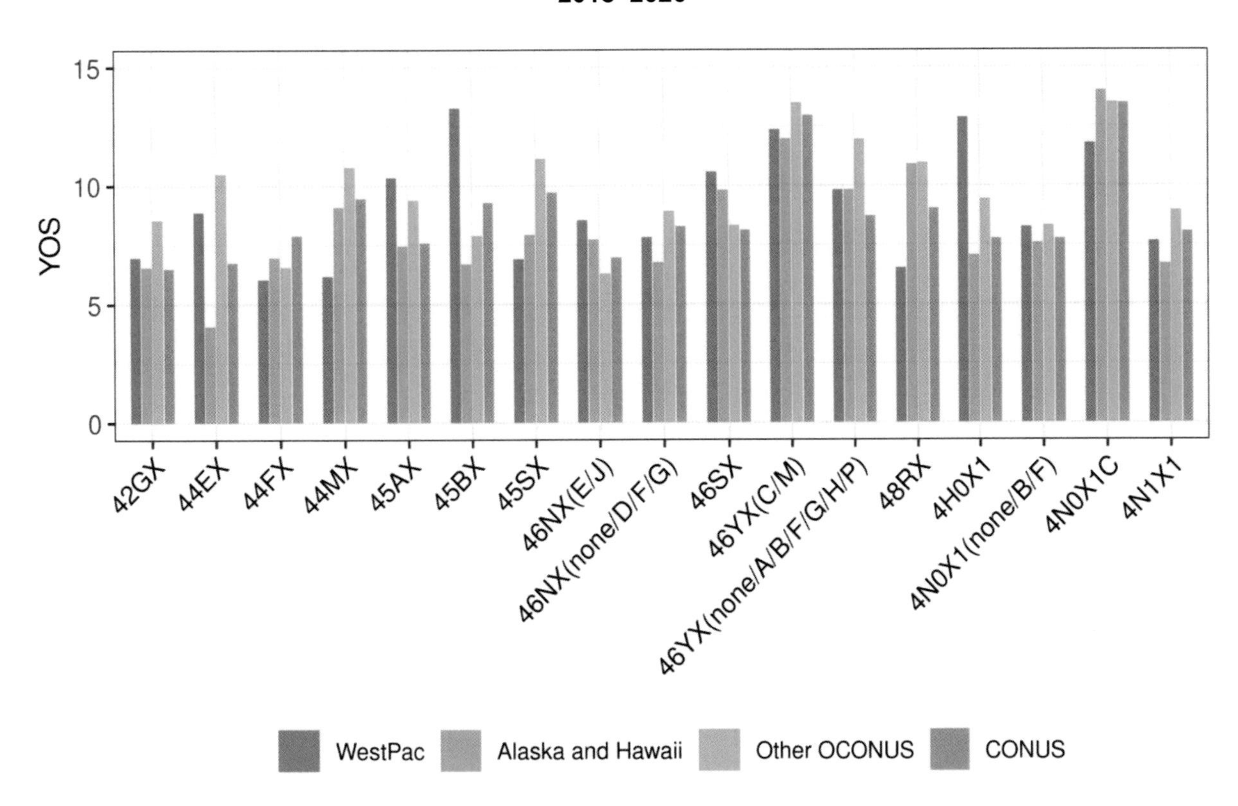

Grade distribution is another measure of experience level. In Figure 2.5, we combined officer ranks into company grade (O-1 to O-3) and field grade (O-4 to O-6) for the 13 officer AFSC groupings. For the entire officer corps in critical medical specialties, the percentage of field-grade officers was highest at WestPac locations (60 percent), followed by Alaska and Hawaii locations (58 percent), CONUS locations (53 percent), and other OCONUS locations

[10] To estimate these values, we performed a logistic regression treating YOS as the outcome and AFSC and location as the predictor variables. The marginal change in YOS associated with being stationed in WestPac, Alaska and Hawaii, OCONUS, and CONUS equaled –0.1, –0.6, 0.8 and –0.2 years, respectively. In other words, individuals assigned to OCONUS locations (other than WestPac and Alaska and Hawaii) had about one more year of experience on average, and individuals assigned to Alaska and Hawaii locations had about 0.6 fewer years of experience on average.

Figure 2.5. Seniority of Officers by Location, 2018–2020

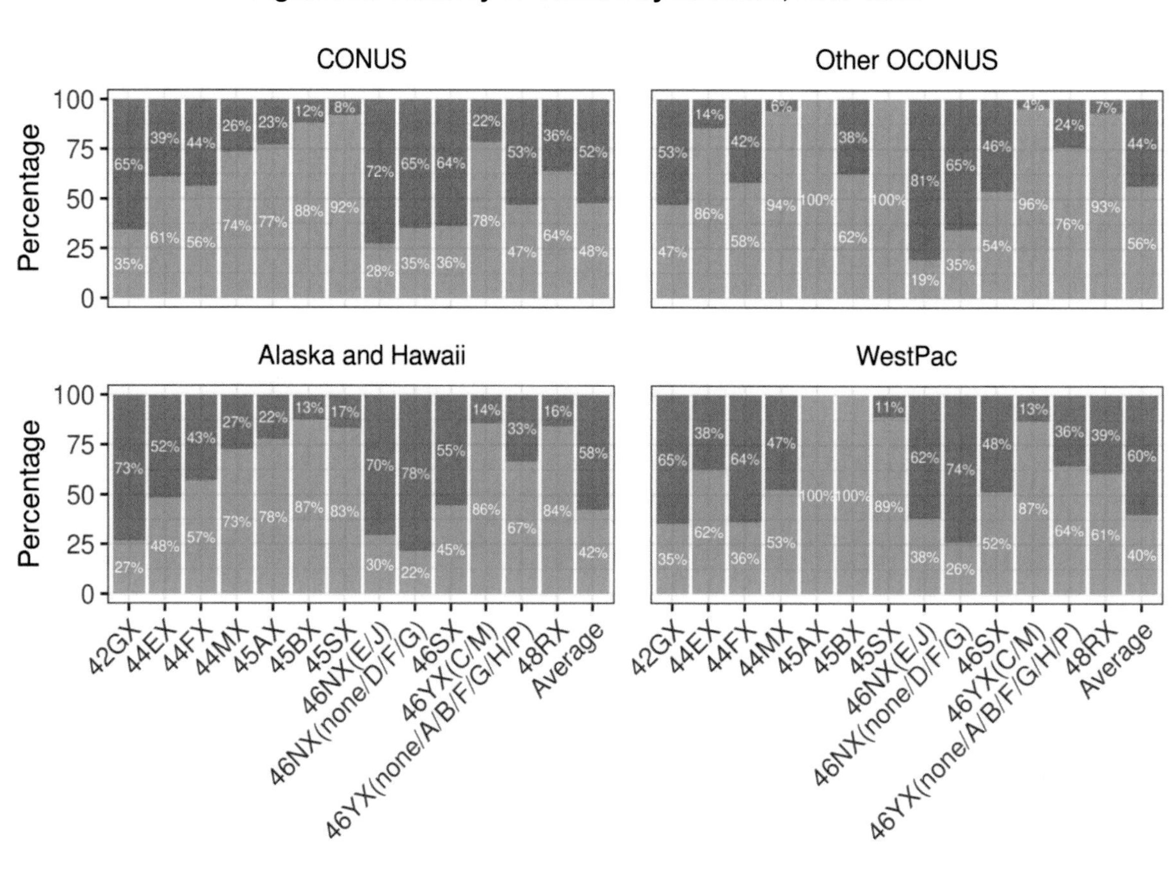

(44 percent). Relatedly, Figure 2.6 shows enlisted grade distributions for the four AFSC groupings and location. We combined enlisted ranks into airman (E-1 to E-4), noncommissioned officer (NCO; E-5 to E-6) and senior NCOs (E-7 to E-9). For all enlisted personnel in critical medical AFSCs, the percentage of NCOs and senior NCOs was greatest at other OCONUS locations (69 percent), followed by WestPac locations (64 percent), and Alaska and Hawaii and CONUS locations (56 percent each).

As a final measure of experience, we analyzed the skill levels of enlisted personnel by location and career field. Enlisted personnel begin their careers at skill level 1 (helper). Upon graduating from technical school, they advance to skill level 3 (apprentice). Airmen go on to skill level 5 (journeyman), skill level 7 (craftsman), and skill level 9 (superintendent) as they

Figure 2.6. Seniority of Enlisted Personnel by Location, 2018–2020

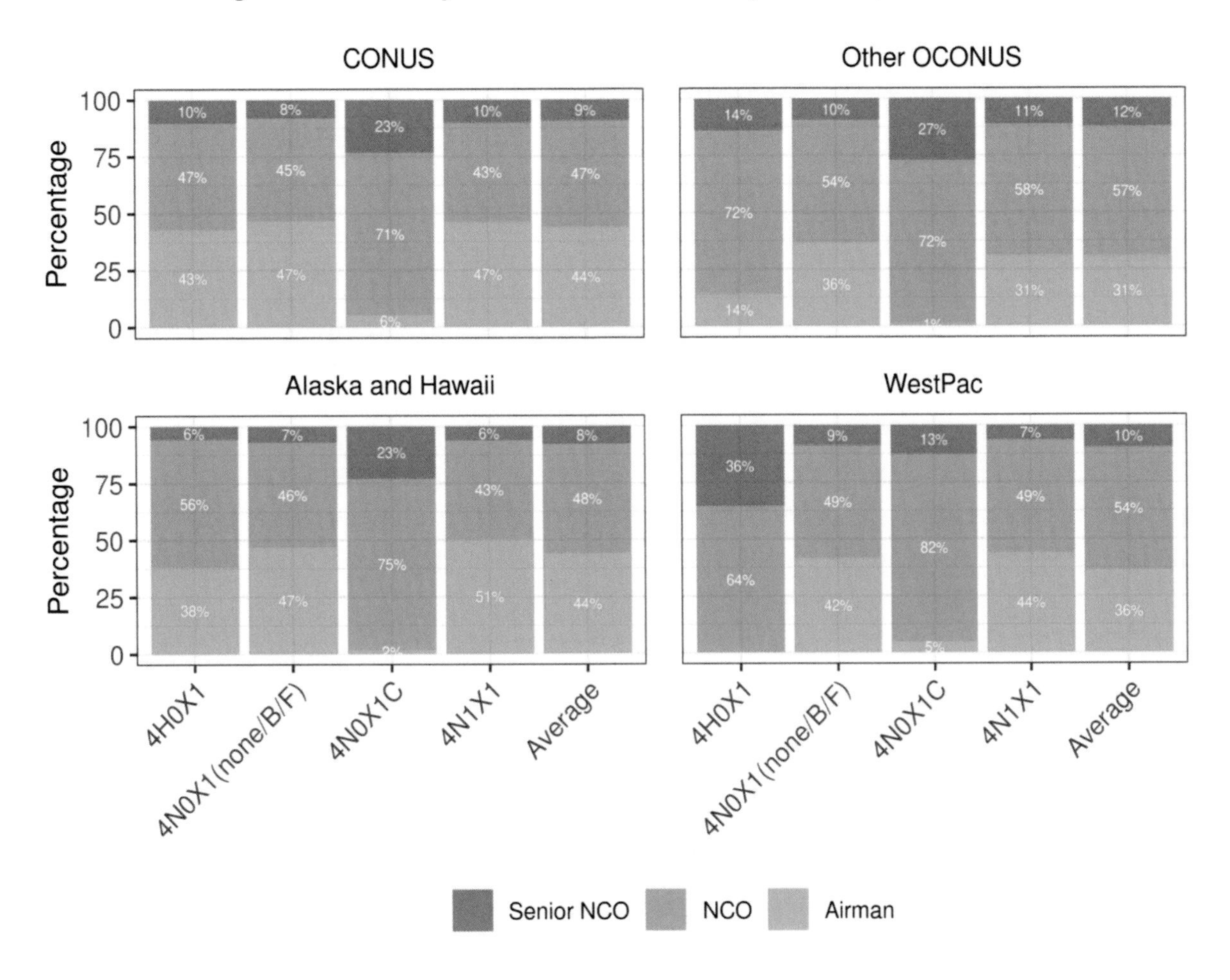

complete additional training and advance through the enlisted ranks. Figure 2.7 shows the percentages of enlisted individuals by skill level and location. For all enlisted personnel in critical medical AFSCs, the number of individuals at skill level 7 or higher was somewhat greater at other OCONUS locations (67 percent) than at WestPac locations (60 percent) or Alaska and Hawaii locations (52 percent). The number was lowest at CONUS locations (52 percent). The number of individuals at skill level 5 or higher was equal for other OCONUS and WestPac locations (92 percent), and it was lower at CONUS (87 percent) and Alaska and Hawaii locations (86 percent).

Figure 2.7. Enlisted Skill Level by Air Force Specialty Code and Location, 2018–2020

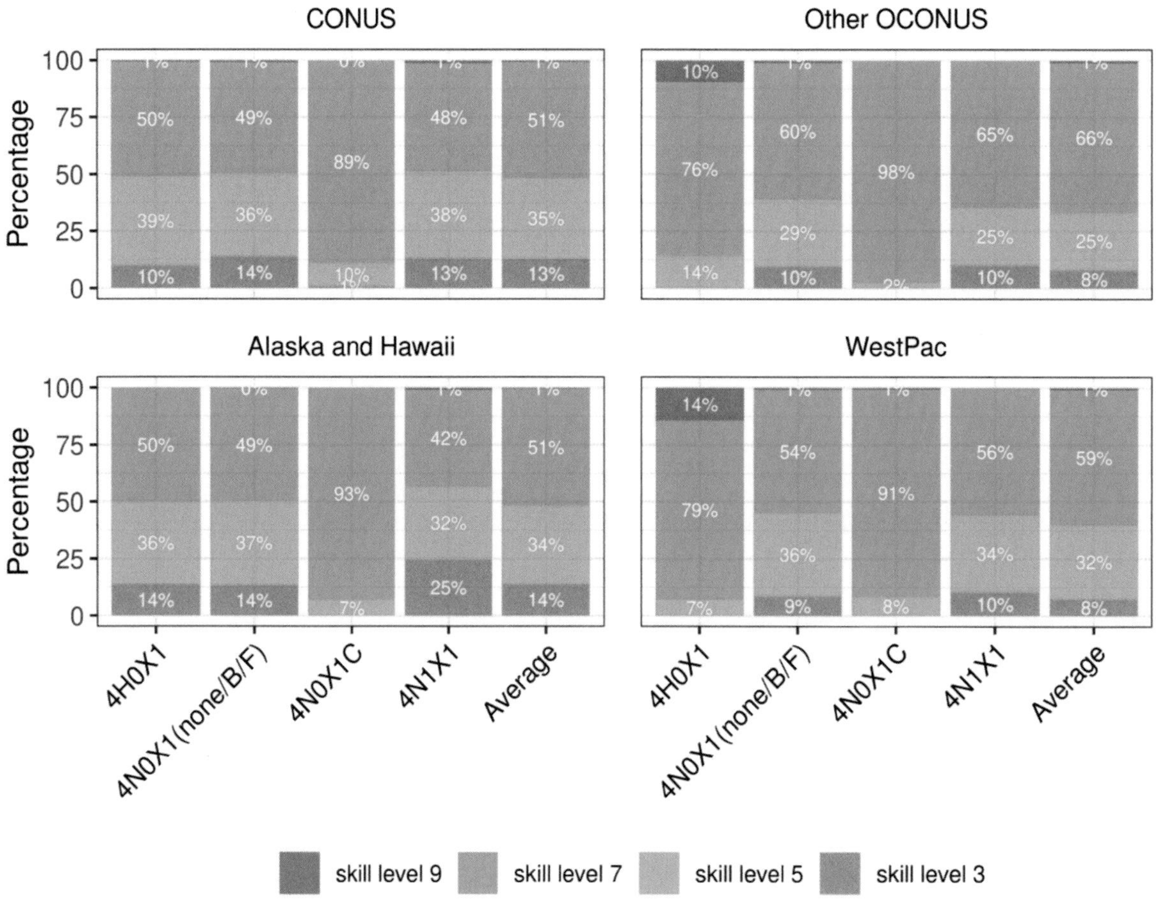

Deployment Tempo by Air Force Specialty Code

Deployment rates for each AFSC are calculated as the average percentage of person-years for each AFSC that are spent deployed from all locations from FY 2018 through FY 2020. As Figure 2.8 shows, deployment rates are lowest for several Advanced Practice Registered Nurses specialties, 46YX(A/B/G/H/P), with an average rate below 1 percent. A little under half of the AFSC groupings have an average deployment rate below an average rate of two weeks a year, as indicated by the dotted line. Several AFSCs have rates above 6 percent, but specialty groups with the highest deployment rates, just above 8 percent (about four weeks a year), are Critical Care and Emergency/Trauma Clinical Nurses, 46NX(E/J), and Acute Care Nurse Practitioners and Certified Registered Nurse Anesthetists, 46Y(C/M). While Family Physicians, 44FX, deploy at a somewhat lower rate than Emergency Services Physicians, 44EX, Anesthesiologists, 45AX, or Surgeons, 45SX, given that they are the largest physician AFSCs, they still represent a large number of deployments overall.

Figure 2.8. Deployment Rates by Air Force Specialty Code, 2018–2020

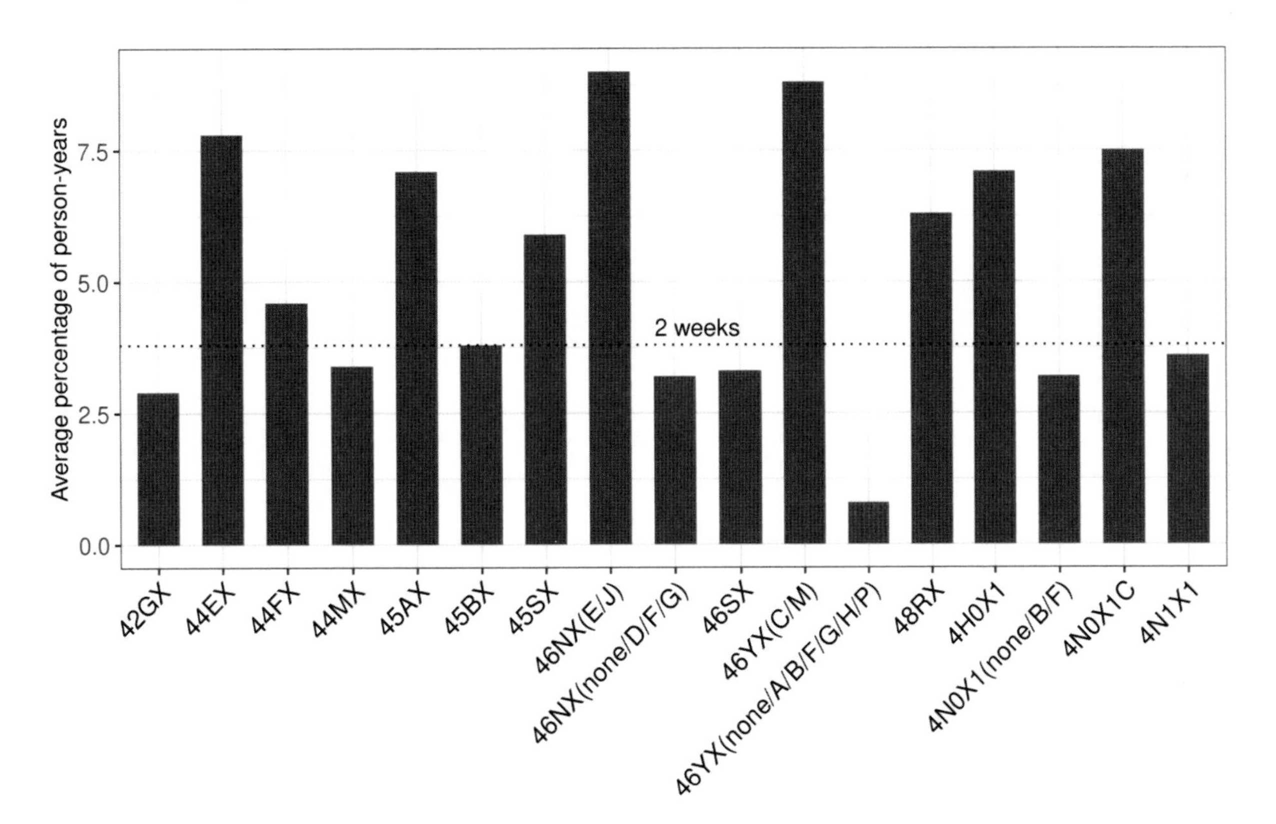

Summary of Manpower and Personnel Analysis

The Air Force prioritizes manning at overseas locations, and our analysis confirms that PACAF does receive slightly more than its fair share of total personnel and experienced personnel as compared with the rest of the Air Force. However, there are relatively few personnel in critical medical specialties assigned to WestPac locations, and some specialties are undermanned. Further, deployments from any location are, on average, likely limited in the contributions they make to overall readiness. More specifically, our analysis can be summarized as follows:

- The number of individuals within each AFSC varies by several orders of magnitude (e.g., from more than 5,000 individuals in Aerospace Medical Service, 4N0X1, to tens of individuals in Emergency Services Physicians, 44EX, and surgical specialties). Such large variations will affect the feasibility of different approaches for building and sustaining clinical proficiency, a point that we return to in Chapters 3 and 4.
- Many specialties are undermanned or critically undermanned. Although undermanning is more common at CONUS locations, certain AFSCs are also undermanned at WestPac, Alaska and Hawaii, and other OCONUS locations. Increasing manning levels will increase the capacity of the AFMS to provide clinical care at undermanned locations.
- Experience levels, measured by YOS, grade distributions, and enlisted skill levels (but not adjusted for time from last high-volume clinical assignment), tended to be lower at CONUS locations than at OCONUS locations (including WestPac and Alaska and Hawaii). Experience levels were also somewhat lower at Alaska and Hawaii locations

than at WestPac locations. This indicates that individuals at Alaska and Hawaii locations may be less ready to provide clinical care.

- Deployment tempo varies widely across AFSCs and within AFSCs by specialty; in fact, the greatest difference in deployment rates was within an AFSC—Advanced Practice Registered Nurses, 46YX. The majority of critical AFSCs were deployed for less than 5 percent of their total time served during the three-year period from 2018 through 2020. This may indicate an even broader gap in time since the last wartime proficiency for personnel in these AFSCs.

Readiness Requirements

The manning and experience levels of medical professionals in different locations represent only one component of the AFMS's ability to provide wartime care; another critical component is the readiness of these personnel in terms of knowledge and skills. To understand the Air Force's medical readiness requirements for each AFSC in this study, and to understand the Air Force's system for monitoring whether medical personnel have met the requirements, we analyzed CMRP checklists for each critical AFSC. In addition, we describe the KSA metric, a recently piloted and noteworthy initiative to assess and improve readiness.

Comprehensive Medical Readiness Program Checklists

CMRP checklists identify the knowledge and skills that personnel in each AFSC must possess and maintain to be qualified to provide in-garrison care and be ready for combat. The checklists include requirements in four categories:

1. *clinical currency*, which includes requirements that focus on knowledge and skills necessary to provide in-garrison care for a given AFSC
2. *readiness skills training*, which includes requirements that relate more to ensuring readiness to provide care in deployed wartime environments for a given AFSC
3. *unit type code training*, which are requirements specific to a unit type code that ensure that a code as a whole has the knowledge and skills to accomplish its mission
4. *installation medical all-hazard response training*, which are requirements pertaining to hazard response equipment, hazardous materials response, and respiratory protection.[11]

We focused our analyses on categories 1 and 2 because they relate most to trauma and critical care skills that decay over time; we considered categories 3 and 4 as out of scope. Examples of category 1 and 2 requirements include professional licensure and certification, trauma management and life support, knowledge of blast and blunt injury, evaluation and treatment of traumatic brain injury, and knowledge of specific Clinical Practice Guidelines from the Joint Trauma Center.

---

[11] Air Force Instruction 41-106, *Air Force Medical Readiness Program*, Department of the Air Force, July 29, 2020.

A CMRP checklist for a given AFSC is developed and maintained by the specialty consultant and may include a wide variety of requirements, some of which involve direct patient care and some of which do not. A clinician may be required to work a minimum number of hours in an emergency department or intensive care unit; perform a given number of specific procedures, such as airway management or evaluation of patients with traumatic brain injury; complete topical courses in person or online; or independently study online documents and videos. Specialty consultants, corps directors, and career field managers develop category 1 and 2 requirements. Per Air Force Instruction 41-106, medical unit commanders or their designees submit information on personnel readiness to the Medical Resource Decision Support System (MRDSS), "the official system of record for the management of expeditionary medical personnel and readiness resources for the AFMS." The MRDSS enables a "gap analysis," which is reviewed on a quarterly basis by specialty consultants, corps directors, and career field managers to identify new or modify existing training programs to mitigate identifiable deficiencies.[12]

Analysis of Comprehensive Medical Readiness Program Checklists

For all critical AFSCs, we systematically reviewed CMRPs, extracted information from each CMRP checklist, and compared requirements on the following dimensions: hours of practice in a specific care setting, such as outpatient, emergency department, inpatient, trauma center, or critical care unit; procedures to be performed, including number and type; and knowledge, including topical areas and formal coursework or self-study to be completed. Two reviewers independently read all CMRP checklists and maintained notes on the dimensions and features of each checklist that stood out as potentially inadequate or incomplete statements of requirements for monitoring and maintaining the readiness of medical personnel.

Project team members discussed reviewers' areas of agreement and disagreement on standout features within each checklist and across multiple checklists. Team members then met with RAND subject-matter experts to discuss these standout features and validated findings during interviews with AFMS stakeholders. Our analysis focused on potential problems with detail, clarity, and usability of CMRP checklists; we did not seek to identify deficits in topical areas of knowledge or skill listed in checklists, though we noted areas where requirements appeared low compared with common standards for medical professions.

Overall, we found wide variation in the intensity of CMRP requirements and unclear communication of requirements in some CMRPs that may make it difficult for the AFMS to track the readiness of medical providers and ensure they are ready to provide wartime care. The six weaknesses in CMRPs we identified are described below.

---

[12] Air Force Instruction 41-106, 2020.

Variation in Number and Intensity of Requirements Suggests Missing Requirements

CMRP checklists vary substantially on the number of requirements they contain and the balance of direct patient care experience, coursework, and self-study they require. For example, the checklist for Surgeon, 45SX, contains a relatively small number of experience and knowledge requirements. The checklist includes a specific number of procedures to be performed, though types of procedures are unspecified in the checklist; a specific number of critical care encounters or hours of practice in a trauma or critical care setting; and knowledge of Clinical Practice Guidelines, though specific guidelines are not listed in the checklist.

In contrast, the Physician Assistant, 42GX, checklist requires hours in multiple types of care settings; procedures, including inpatient or outpatient procedures, evaluation, and treatment of patients with traumatic brain injury and evaluation of patients with combat stress; and an extensive list of courses, such as the Air Force Physician Assistant Refresher Course and Global Medicine Course. The Clinical Nurse, 46NX, checklist requires a specific number of hours in a trauma center and knowledge of many clinical practice guidelines but no specific procedures or coursework. While we would expect requirements to vary by specialty, these differences suggest that the CMRP checklists for some specialties are not comprehensive and provide a less than adequate method for judging currency and readiness. Opportunities may exist to achieve better balance of readiness activities for some specialties.

Variation in Wartime-Specific Requirements Suggests Missing Requirements

While readiness for wartime is a priority for all medical personnel, only some CMRP checklists reference knowledge and skills specific to wartime. For example, checklists for Physician Assistant, 42GX, and Aerospace Medical Service, 4N0X1, require knowledge and coursework specific to wartime, such as blast injury and in-theater patient movement, while most physician checklists lack reference to activities specifically tailored to practicing in wartime environments. This again suggests that readiness requirements are not fully stated in CMRP checklists even though these checklists are the method by which readiness is assessed for the individual, the unit, and the specialty.

Low and Potentially Insufficient Patient Care Hours Requirements

Required patient care hours for some AFSCs appear low.[13] For example, the CMRP checklist for Operating Room Nurse, 46SX, requires a minimum performance of only 24 hours annually as a surgical scrub nurse. In contrast, a registered nurse must have at least 1,200 hours of surgical experience to be eligible for the Certified Perioperative Nurse credential from the Competency and Credentialing Institute.[14] This civilian benchmark suggests that 24 hours annually is

---

[13] Commander at Brooke Army Medical Center, interview with the authors, April 27, 2021; former medical group commander, interview with the authors, July 16, 2021.

[14] Competency and Credentialing Institute, "Certified Perioperative Nurse," webpage, undated.

insufficient to maintain clinical currency and readiness to support an operating room during wartime.

Options for Meeting Patient-Care Hours May Not Offer Equivalent Readiness

To meet requirements for hours of experiences, CMRP checklists state that medical personnel may work in various clinical settings, including MTFs, civilian facilities with special agreements to host military health care providers, a Center for the Sustainment of Trauma and Readiness Skills (C-STARS) site, a Sustained Medical and Readiness Trained (SMART) Regional Currency Site, and "moonlighting" in off-duty employment (ODE). Trauma centers and certain high-acuity civilian hospitals likely provide better preparation for wartime than MTFs because they consistently care for a higher volume of trauma and critical care patients who require emergency resuscitation.[15] However, the checklists do not sufficiently capture expected differences in readiness generated by these activities, nor do they direct medical personnel to complete their hours with options that best improve readiness.

Unclear Communication of Requirements

Some checklists lack the specificity that may be needed to communicate readiness requirements and determine whether they are being met. For example, some checklists require personnel to perform specific procedures each year but do not specify the number of procedures. Others list multiple activities needed to stay current on a given topic—such as courses to be taken at one-, two-, or four-year intervals—but do not specify whether *any* or *all* activities must be completed to meet the requirement. This lack of clarity contributes to a perception that personnel who have not fully met all requirements can nevertheless self-report as having fulfilled the CMRP checklist and face minimal accountability.[16] This lack of clarity can contribute to unclear assessments of the readiness of an individual or unit.

The Knowledge, Skills, and Abilities Metric Under Development

A noteworthy initiative to develop and assess the clinical KSAs needed in wartime is the DoD's Clinical Readiness Program,[17] which includes the use of a KSA metric to measure a provider's clinical currency and competency. The metric is calculated based on the number and type of procedures performed by an individual over the preceding 12 months, recorded using procedural terminology codes at an MTF or other setting. Each procedure is assigned a point value based on factors such as clinical complexity. The point value corresponds to KSAs

---

[15] Berwick, Downey, and Cornett, 2016, p. 99.

[16] Current medical group commander, interview with the authors, May 6, 2021; former medical group commander, interview with the authors, July 16, 2021.

[17] Danielle B. Holt, Matthew T. Hueman, Jonathan Jaffin, Michael Sanchez, Mark A. Hamilton, Charles D. Mabry, Jeffrey A. Bailey, and Eric A. Elster, "Clinical Readiness Program: Refocusing the Military Health System," *Military Medicine*, Vol. 186, No. 1, January 25, 2021.

required to provide care in deployed settings, as determined by military medical subject-matter experts. Examples of procedures contributing points toward KSA scores include torso trauma operations, transfusion and resuscitation, and airway and breathing care. Points are then aggregated to produce scores that apply to specific time periods, and they are adjusted by predefined factors (e.g., diversity score, complexity discount) before they are used to compare scores across providers.[18]

Developers of the KSA score convened expert panel discussions and reviewed case registries and recent scholarship to validate scores, thresholds, and limitations of KSA scoring. Based on discussions with DoD subject-matter experts, the KSA score appears to be a promising means of assessing clinical currency for providers who are required to perform a certain number of procedures (e.g., general and orthopedic surgeons). Providers would be responsible for recording the number of qualifying procedures to monitor their progress toward the readiness threshold.[19]

DoD began testing the KSA metric for general surgeons and orthopedic surgeons at six MTFs in 2018, with plans to expand to other provider specialties and use the metric to determine whether additional training may be needed prior to deployment.[20] As outlined, the KSA metric could be used in conjunction with provider-specific CMRP checklists to better understand readiness for medical personnel across the AFMS.

However, three issues described in a U.S. Government Accountability Office report are likely to prevent rapid adoption and complete replacement of existing readiness evaluation tools: (1) at present, the KSA score does not account for procedures done outside an MTF; (2) provider clinical case mix at MTFs is not likely to approximate that of deployed providers; and (3) while the KSA metric reflects the number and type of procedures that providers perform, the ability to meet a KSA threshold does not provide any information about patient safety and clinical outcomes, especially in an austere environment. An additional concern is that the KSAs have not been validated as reliably predicting clinical proficiency in deployed medical and surgical skills.

Furthermore, during our discussions with DoD subject-matter experts, they voiced three additional limitations of the KSA score that may limit its validity: (1) current methods can produce obvious outliers for personnel whose names may be listed on case logs even if they were not present (i.e., in the event that the department chair is always listed); (2) scores may be more useful for evaluating group performance than for comparing performance among individuals due to idiosyncrasies in practice variation and procedure coding; and (3) reliance on procedure counts may not be a valid assessment of performance for professionals who rarely need to perform procedures (e.g., general internists).

---

[18] Uniformed Services University, "Clinical Readiness Program: Combat Casualty Care KSAs," briefing, April 2018.

[19] Uniformed Services University, 2018.

[20] U.S. Government Accountability Office, *Defense Health Care: Actions Needed to Determine the Size and Readiness of Operational Medical and Dental Forces*, GAO-19-206, February 2019.

Summary of Readiness Requirements Analysis

The AFMS uses CMRP checklists to identify readiness requirements for medical professionals—such as requirements to practice for a specific number of hours in certain settings, perform a specific number and type of procedures, and complete formal courses or self-study—and evaluate the readiness of medical professionals to provide care in wartime. Currently, multiple weaknesses of the checklists may make it difficult to track the readiness of medical providers at the individual level and in aggregate through the MRDSS.[21]

As an initial step toward improving readiness, the AFMS could improve the checklists by increasing the specificity and consistency of requirements across checklists. This step could help AFMS personnel tasked with monitoring and ensuring readiness to collect data on the extent to which CMRP requirements are being met. In addition, the AFMS could incorporate the KSA metric recently piloted by DoD into the CMRP checklists. However, improvements in data and refinement of methods may be needed before the KSA metric can be usefully incorporated.

Our review of CMRP checklists suggests that the U.S. Air Force could improve clinical readiness and its tracking by increasing the specificity and consistency across CMRPs. These improvements could ultimately enable improved identification of gaps in clinical readiness so that any shortfalls can be addressed prior to deployment or assignment to WestPac. Currently, those tasked with monitoring and ensuring readiness are using checklists that do not allow for clear identification of gaps in the knowledge and skills needed to ensure the best outcomes for personnel injured in combat or treated at a home station.

Beyond improving manning levels and monitoring of AFMS personnel readiness, multiple options exist for improving readiness. Chapters 3 and 4 describe these options in detail.

---

[21] Former medical group commander, interview with the authors, July 16, 2021.

Chapter 3. Readiness Building: Training and Practice Activities

Current methods to assess medical readiness fall short in identifying the type and volume of activities military medical professionals need to be engaged in to maintain clinical proficiency and be ready to respond to trauma during wartime. As discussed in the previous chapters, there is a disconnect between the clinical care that professionals are providing during peacetime assignments and the trauma-related skills they will need to provide high-quality care during active conflicts. To help resolve this disconnect, we identified a set of activities to help enhance and maintain medical readiness for personnel in critical medical specialties, which we describe in this chapter.

To identify these readiness building activities, we considered "building blocks" of readiness discussed in previous research,[1] which included a range of activities, from education and training courses; to opportunities to work in facilities outside an MTF for additional clinical experience, such as civilian trauma centers or U.S. Department of Veterans Affairs (VA) Veterans Affairs Medical Centers (VAMCs); to sequencing of assignments that enable more varied practice opportunities over time. We additionally relied on readiness activities listed in CMRP checklists for critical AFSCs, such as practice requirements in specific settings and formal coursework.

After establishing a candidate list of readiness activities, we reviewed evidence about the impact of each activity from peer-reviewed and gray literature. In addition, we conducted semistructured interviews with a sample of key informants to learn more about the perceived impacts and implementation challenges of each activity. The sample consisted of AFMS leadership, including the PACAF surgeon general and his staff; individuals who currently serve or recently served in PACAF, including medical professionals within MTFs, Critical Care Air Transport Teams, and Special Operations Surgical Teams, and at Brooke Army Medical Center; and individuals responsible for training AFMS medical professionals, including instructors at the U.S. Air Force School of Aerospace Medicine (USAFSAM) and C-STARS sites.

With the information obtained from the literature review and the interviews, we compiled a comprehensive set of 15 readiness building activities and policies, listed in Table 3.1, which fall into three categories: training activities, practice activities, and assignment policies, as introduced in Chapter 1. *Training* activities encompass didactic education that may or may not include hands-on experience, such as precepted (instructor-supervised) patient care and/or simulated patient care. *Practice* activities offer opportunities to provide nonprecepted direct patient care for trauma or other critical care patients that improves wartime medical knowledge and performance of key procedures. *Assignment* policies tailor the order, length, or location of a medical provider's assignments to help maintain and improve wartime knowledge and performance.

---

[1] Chan, Krull, Ahluwalia, Broyles, Waxman, Gurvey, Colthirst, Schimmels, and Marinos, 2020.

Table 3.1. Readiness Building Activities and Policies

Category	Readiness Activity or Policy
Training activities	• Attending C-STARS before or during PACAF assignment • Attending a trauma training course • Attend advanced simulation training
Practice activities	• Practicing in a trauma center MTF • Practicing intermittently at higher-volume MTF via a temporary duty (TDY) within-skill exchange program • Embedding at a civilian Level 1 trauma center • Embedding at a civilian Level 1 trauma center as members of the C-STARS cadre • Practicing intermittently at a civilian Level 1 trauma center • Embedding at a VAMC • Embedding at a VAMC as a cadre • Practicing intermittently at a VAMC • Using off-duty-employment to practice intermittently at civilian trauma center or intensive care unit
Assignment policies	• Reducing tour lengths at low-volume locations • Sequencing assignments to maintain or increase proficiency • Using military workforce at high-volume locations and nonmilitary workforce at low-volume locations

Within and across categories, the readiness activities and policies vary on multiple dimensions, including duration, whether they are designed for individuals or teams, the mix of direct patient care and formal instruction they require, the type of care setting within which they are conducted, the patient population they involve, and the costs involved.

The remainder of this chapter describes the actions the Air Force could take to implement or expand these readiness building activities in the training and practice categories. We do not expect the Air Force to implement all of these training and practice activities; they are presented as a broad menu of potential options that could be adopted to enhance readiness, either on their own or in combination. Chapter 4 discusses assignment policies and associated analyses.

Training Activities

Readiness activities in the training category include sending medical professionals to C-STARS before deployment to PACAF; implementation of a novel traveling trauma course program; and increased investment in simulation or other training technology to improve access to training at MTFs and other locations where medical professionals practice during peacetime.

Mandating Training at C-STARS Before or During Pacific Air Forces Assignment

In this activity, all personnel within targeted AFSCs would attend trauma training at C-STARS in preparation for forward assignment or midway through forward assignment. C-STARS is a two-week program in trauma care that combines classroom instruction, simulation training, and on-the-job training through patient care at three locations. C-STARS fulfills many of the requirements listed in the CMRPs for targeted AFSCs; in fact, the CMRPs often reference C-STARS as a pathway to meet the requirements. A precedent exists for using C-STARS to provide predeployment and middeployment training, as C-STARS was often used for predeployment training for the wars in Afghanistan and Iraq and some Air Force personnel have attended C-STARS training while assigned to PACAF overseas bases.[2] Notably, this activity (i.e., increasing the number of C-STARS *trainees*) differs from increasing the number of C-STARS cadre members (i.e., *instructors*) described later in this chapter.

The existing C-STARS program appears to have the capacity to accommodate the number of Air Force personnel assigned to PACAF each year, though some adjustment would be needed to implement this activity. The capacity and topical focus of C-STARS sites varies. The C-STARS site at the University of Maryland Medical Center's Shock Trauma Center, the largest C-STARS site, trains an estimated 300 Air Force personnel per year and focuses on trauma and surgical skills.[3]

The site at the University of Cincinnati Medical Center focuses on aeromedical evacuation of critically injured patients and trains an estimated 170 to 210 personnel per year.[4] Air Force Critical Care Air Transport Teams and Tactical Critical Care Evacuation Teams attend the program,[5] with each team consisting of three members who train together: a critical care or emergency doctor, a critical care nurse, and a respiratory technician. The C-STARS site at St. Louis University Hospital trains an estimated 250 Air Force personnel per year and focuses on trauma skills.[6] Our analysis of administrative data available from the USAFSAM education portal indicates that vacancies in C-STARS class seats would accommodate the number of Air Force personnel assigned to PACAF each year, though less slack exists for some AFSCs, and the number of slots would need to be adjusted among AFSCs.

Overall, the history of using C-STARS for predeployment and middeployment training and the existing capacity to accommodate the number of Air Force personnel assigned to PACAF make this activity attractive for helping Air Force medical personnel meet CMRP requirements and improve their readiness. Mandating C-STARS to accommodate all personnel assigned to

---

[2] Chad M. Thorson, Joseph J. Dubose, Peter Rhee, Thomas E. Knuth, Warren C. Dorlac, Jeffrey A. Bailey, George D. Garcia, Mark L. Ryan, Robert M. Van Haren, and Kenneth G. Proctor, "Military Trauma Training at Civilian Centers: A Decade of Advancements," *Journal of Trauma and Acute Care Surgery*, Vol. 73, No. 6, December 2012; Cannon, Gross, and Rasmussen, 2020.

[3] Deputy Group Commander Chief Nurse, "Sustained Medical & Readiness Trained (SMART)," 6th Medical Group, briefing, undated. The site trains approximately 30 Air Force personnel per month; University of Maryland School of Medicine, "C-STARS (Center for the Sustainment of Trauma and Readiness Skills)," webpage, undated.

[4] University of Cincinnati Medical Center, "C-STARS Simulation Center Helps U.S. Air Force Medical Personnel Train," webpage, undated. The site conducts 14 classes per year, with 12 to 15 Air Force personnel per class; UC Health, "C-STARS: University of Cincinnati Medical Center Cincinnati C-STARS," webpage, undated.

[5] Marisa Alia-Novobilski, "C-STARS Visit Highlights Trauma Training," Air Force Medical Service, June 19, 2018.

[6] Deputy Group Commander Chief Nurse, undated. The site trained more than 4,000 Air Force medical personnel from 2003 to 2018; Kathleen Nelson, "SSM Health Hospital Trains Military Medical Personnel Headed to Combat Zones," Catholic Health Association of the United States, April 15, 2018.

WestPac would provide real-life experience with trauma care, an important component of readiness. Travel to a C-STARS location and time away from home and family could impose costs on trainees, though the change of environment and daily tasks involved in attending C-STARS could also benefit them. For the Air Force and its MTFs, this activity would entail travel costs and could require backfilling positions while personnel attend C-STARS in order to avoid disruption in patient care at MTFs.

There are, on average, 247 permanent change-of-station moves to WestPac locations annually for airmen in critical medical specialties. Two weeks of C-STARS training, plus two days for travel, amounts to a manpower cost of close to 11 full-time equivalent (FTE) personnel and travel costs of approximately $687,000 annually.[7] This estimate assumes that all individuals being assigned to WestPac attend; however, some personnel may have already attended recently. PACAF could also decide to prioritize some specialties over others within a fixed manpower and dollar allocation. However, travel costs would be higher for personnel who travel to C-STARS from WestPac locations midway through deployment than for personnel who travel to C-STARS from other CONUS locations prior to PACAF deployment. This activity would not significantly benefit the civilian trauma centers that host C-STARS programs, since trauma centers derive the most benefit from a cadre that can provide substantial amounts of patient care.

Developing a Traveling Trauma Course

Air Force medical personnel located in WestPac could be offered a readiness-generating activity via a traveling trauma course program. We envision that a multidisciplinary team of approximately five instructors would do a yearly tour to provide interactive classroom instruction and host team-based simulation activities at each of the six WestPac MTFs.[8] Course content would be designed to enhance trauma knowledge and performance, and it could include content from preexisting courses such as Brigade Combat Team Trauma Training, Tactical Combat Medical Care, Surgical Team Assessment Training, Chemical/Biological Casualty, Combat Casualty, Advanced Trauma Life Support, Advanced Burn Life Support, Combat Stress Casualty, Emergency War Surgery, and/or Combat Extremity Surgery.[9] To our knowledge, a traveling trauma course is not currently offered to Air Force medical personnel in WestPac;

---

[7] This estimate assumes an average per diem of $155 for 16 days and airfare of $300 per attendee; U.S. General Services Administration, "FY 2023 Per Diem Highlights," webpage, August, 12, 2021.

[8] The composition of the team could be scaled up or down depending on the expected number and skills of the attendees. Discussions with subject-matter experts suggested that a typical training team could comprise one physician, one nurse, one operating room technician, one IDMT, and one additional technician.

[9] Martin Meiners, "JBSA–Fort Sam Houston Experts Provide Fort Campbell Medics Brigade Combat Team Trauma Training," Joint Base San Antonio, March 21, 2017; Rebecca Westfall, "Tactical Combat Medical Care Course Hones Combat Medical Readiness," U.S. Army, May 6, 2019; Dwight C. Kellicut, Eric J. Kuncir, Hope M. Williamson, Pamela C. Masella, and Peter E. Nielsen, "Surgical Team Assessment Training: Improving Surgical Teams During Deployment," *American Journal of Surgery*, Vol. 208, No. 2, May 2014; U.S. Army Medical Department and School, U.S. Army Health Readiness Center of Excellence, *Course Catalog 2018*, Joint Base San Antonio, August 2017.

however, there is precedent for conducting traveling trauma courses in Army surgical resuscitation medical treatment facilities in Iraq, so a similar program for PACAF medical personnel could be launched.[10]

Most or all medical personnel, across a range of specialties, at WestPac MTFs could participate in a traveling trauma course, which would focus on developing both individual and team-based skills in trauma care. Current evidence suggests that improving teamwork leads to improved outcomes for patients and that simulations of procedural skills can lead to a reduction in patient safety problems.[11] While options to enhance trauma team skills exist for medical personnel in WestPac (e.g., traveling to a C-STARS or SMART site in CONUS), these options are time- and resource-intensive for individuals whose primary duty is in an MTF. A traveling trauma course would enable WestPac personnel to sharpen knowledge and trauma team skills under the instruction of experienced instructors without having to leave their MTFs.

The traveling trauma course could last between two and five days at each site, depending on resource availability and the ability of MTFs to sustain routine practice activities while excusing a portion of the medical staff to participate in the course. Traveling trauma course instructors could be drawn from a pool of experienced medical personnel with assignments in CONUS, such as those actively practicing at C-STARS and SMART sites. Alternatively, instructors could be medical personnel with experience practicing medicine in deployed environments. Instructors could travel with simulation equipment that is more advanced than equipment currently available at most MTFs in WestPac.

A traveling trauma course would enhance readiness—particularly for personnel located at facilities that care for the fewest trauma and critical care patients, such as those at Kunsan Air Base and Osan Air Base. This readiness-generating activity would be designed to enhance team-based performance during simulated trauma resuscitation and management activities. Given the parameters provided previously, the manpower cost for instructors is estimated to be a maximum of approximately 0.8 FTEs (i.e., three five-day courses per month for two months for each instructor absent from his or her assigned MTF) and travel costs of approximately $55,500

---

[10] Kellicut, Kuncir, Williamson, Masella, and Nielsen, 2014.

[11] Daniel L. Davenport, William G. Henderson, Cecilia L. Mosca, Shukri F. Khuri, and Robert M. Mentzer, Jr., "Risk-Adjusted Morbidity in Teaching Hospitals Correlates with Reported Levels of Communication and Collaboration on Surgical Teams but Not with Scale Measures of Teamwork Climate, Safety Climate, or Working Conditions," *Journal of American College of Surgeons*, Vol. 205, No. 6, December 2007; Karen Mazzocco, Diana B. Petitti, Kenneth T. Fong, Doug Bonacum, John Brookey, Suzanne Graham, Robert E. Lasky, J. Bryan Sexton, and Eric J. Thomas, "Surgical Team Behaviors and Patient Outcomes," *American Journal of Surgery*, Vol. 197, No. 5, May 2009; Teodor P. Grantcharov, Viggo B. Kristiansen, Jørgen Bendix, Linda Bardram, Jacob Rosenberg, and Peter Funch-Jensen, "Randomized Clinical Trial of Virtual Reality Simulation for Laparoscopic Skills Training," *British Journal of Surgery*, Vol. 91, No. 2, February 2004; Gunnar Ahlberg, Lars Enochsson, Anthony G. Gallagher, Leif Hedman, Christian Hogman, David A. McClusky III, Stig Ramel, C. Daniel Smith, and Dag Arvidsson, "Proficiency-Based Virtual Reality Training Significantly Reduces the Error Rate for Residents During Their First 10 Laparoscopic Cholecystectomies," *American Journal of Surgery*, Vol. 193, No. 6, June 2007.

annually.[12] There are also costs for the time that attendees would be away from their MTF responsibilities. It is unlikely that all of the over 600 personnel in critical medical specialties assigned to WestPac would attend, but if they did, the estimated manpower cost for attendees is a maximum of just over eight FTEs.

Investing in Simulation Training

To enable more medical personnel to attend advanced simulation training, the Air Force would need to accelerate the development of simulation training technology and expand access to simulation training at MTFs. However, deciding how to invest in simulation would require dedicated study, since there is a wide variety of simulation training options; and each option has unique costs, manpower considerations, and potential to improve currency and readiness.

Currently, simulation for medical care encompasses a variety of modes ranging from low-tech box trainers and homemade simulators; to practice on simulated bodies and cadavers; to virtual reality (VR), augmented reality, and mixed reality systems.[13] Reported costs of simulation vary widely (see Appendix B). For example, commercially available and custom-made models for burn escharotomy, emergency department thoracotomy, and extracorporeal CPR range in cost from $75 to tens of thousands of dollars;[14] a one-day "boot camp" with cadaveric trainer stations and other simulations can cost $16,000, while an obstetric emergency training course at a UK hospital can cost €148,806 (~US$170,000) to start up and operate for one year.[15] One review found that hardware for a high-end VR trainer cost £3,000 (~US$4,050), with a software cost of less than one-tenth that of a physical simulation, while another study found that VR systems ranged from about $2,000 to $100,000 or more.[16] For comparison, low-cost flight simulator

---

[12] This estimate assumes an average per diem of $155 for 60 days and airfare for six trips for five instructors at $300 each; U.S. General Services Administration, 2021.

[13] Sarah Hoopes, Truce Pham, Fiona M. Lindo, and Danielle D. Antosh, "Home Surgical Skill Training Resources for Obstetrics and Gynecology Trainees During a Pandemic," *Obstetrics and Gynecology*, Vol. 136, No. 1, July 2020; Brian P. Cervenka, Tsung-yen Hsieh, Sharon Lin, and Arnaud Bewley, "Multi-Institutional Regional Otolaryngology Bootcamp," *Annals of Otology, Rhinology and Laryngology*, Vol. 129, No. 6, June 2020; Ryan Lohre, Jeffrey C. Wang, Kai-Uwe Lewandrowski, and Danny P. Goel, "Virtual Reality in Spinal Endoscopy: A Paradigm Shift in Education to Support Spine Surgeons," *Journal of Spine Surgery*, Vol. 6, No. S1, January 2020.

[14] Irene Y. Zhang, Mark Thomas, Barclay T. Stewart, Eleanor Curtis, Carolyn Blayney, Samuel P. Mandell, Vance Y. Sohn, and Tam N. Pham, "Validation of a Low-Cost Simulation Strategy for Burn Escharotomy Training," *Injury*, Vol. 51, No. 9, September 2020; Deena I. Bengiamin, Cory Toomasian, Dustin D. Smith, and Timothy P. Young, "Emergency Department Thoracotomy: A Cost-Effective Model for Simulation Training," *Journal of Emergency Medicine*, Vol. 57, No. 3, September 2019; G. Pang, C. Futter, J. Pincus, J. Dhanani, and K. B. Laupland, "Development and Testing of a Low Cost Simulation Manikin for Extracorporeal Cardiopulmonary Resuscitation (ECPR) Using 3-Dimensional Printing," *Resuscitation*, Vol. 149, April 2020.

[15] Cervenka, Hsieh, Lin, and Bewley, 2020; Christopher W. H. Yau, Elena Pizzo, Steve Morris, David E. Odd, Cathy Winter, and Timothy J. Draycott, "The Cost of Local, Multi-Professional Obstetric Emergencies Training," *Acta Obstetricia et Gynecologica Scandinavica*, Vol. 95, No. 10, October 2016.

[16] Jack Pottle, "Virtual Reality and the Transformation of Medical Education," *Future Healthcare Journal*, Vol. 6, No. 3, October 2019; Hoopes, Pham, Lindo, and Antosh, 2020.

hardware for the Air Force's Pilot Training Next initiative costs $40,000–$45,000, while traditional flight simulators cost $26 million.[17] VR and similar technologies may reduce costs and increase access to simulation, as compared with simulation modes based on physical equipment.

Over the last few decades, military medical simulation capability has expanded substantially as new technology has emerged. In 2008 the Air Force developed a program to establish and coordinate simulation centers across the globe. The U.S. Navy has introduced simulation training at the unit level so that training can be done even at small MTFs through the use of task trainers and mannequin simulators.[18] In 2021 the U.S. Air Force and U.S. Space Force increased investment in medical simulation programs via $1.5 million in contracts with a VR medical simulation platform called SimX, which is designed to improve operational medical handoffs, allow practice missions involving multiple medical teams, and gain experience providing care under dynamic environmental conditions such as winter storms.[19]

In general, studies of the impact of medical simulation are small in scale and characterized by low quality or design flaws.[20] However, one recent systematic review of literature on simulation for developing surgical skills found simulation-based medical education to be effective for developing and preventing decay of procedural skills in surgery.[21] Implementation of any simulation option is likely to have variable success depending on the level of dedication of its leader, but investing in simulation could be an important strategy for improving readiness at all MTFs, including those in WestPac. Simulation holds promise for improving readiness by increasing access to and reducing costs of training, but more research may be required to determine where to target simulation investments to best improve readiness.

A foundation exists on which to expand the Air Force's use of simulation. Currently, multiple entities within the Air Force develop and manage simulation training. For example, USAFSAM oversees many of the training programs that use simulation, including C-STARS, which uses such real-world simulation modes as advanced mannequins, simulated battlefields,

---

[17] Jamie Hunter, "The Truth About the Air Force's Biggest Changes to Pilot Training Since the Dawn of the Jet Age," *The Drive*, August 3, 2021; Jennifer-Leigh Oprihory, "USAF Brings Pilot Training Next to Regular Training in Experimental Curriculum," *Air and Space Forces Magazine*, March 12, 2020.

[18] Allison A. Eubanks, Keith Volner, and Joseph O. Lopreiato, *Past Present and Future of Simulation in Military Medicine*, Treasure Island, Fla.: StatPearls Publishing, November 14, 2020.

[19] Auganix.org, "SimX Receives New U.S. Air Force Contracts Totaling over $1.5 Million to Advance Virtual Reality Training Programs," May 3, 2021.

[20] Mark Higgins, Christopher Madan, and Rakesh Patel, "Development and Decay of Procedural Skills in Surgery: A Systematic Review of the Effectiveness of Simulation-Based Medical Education Interventions," *The Surgeon*, Vol. 19, No. 4, August 2021; Camille Legoux, Richard Gerein, Kathy Boutis, Nicholas Barrowman, and Amy Plint, "Retention of Critical Procedural Skills After Simulation Training: A Systematic Review," *AEM Education and Training*, Vol. 5, No. 3, July 2021; Lohre, Wang, Lewandrowski, and Goe, 2020.

[21] Higgins, Madan, and Patel, 2021.

and simulated treatment of patients on helicopter flights.[22] Additionally, AFWERX, the Air Force Research Laboratory, and the 24th Special Operations Wing are managing and funding development of the SimX VR medical simulator.[23] Many MTFs, including some PACAF forward locations, have simulation facilities with basic simulation equipment. The Air Force's 911th Air Wing in Pittsburgh partnered with Robert Morris University's Regional Innovation in Simulation Education Center to offer a simulation training curriculum to help meet CMRP requirements for registered nurses and Aerospace Medical Service, 4N0X1, personnel.[24]

Investing in simulation training could help reduce disruptions in patient care associated with some other readiness activities (e.g., requiring WestPac personnel to attend C-STARS during their assignment), though it would still take time away from patient care at MTFs. Simulation training could be tailored to the needs of personnel in targeted AFSCs; it could vary in duration from hours to days, be provided to individuals or teams, and be made more accessible through incorporation into existing trainings (e.g., structured trainings required by the physician assistant CMRP) or permanent provision on-site at MTFs.

As we have noted, expansion of simulation training would also entail costs associated with purchasing or developing new technologies and training personnel to lead simulation activities. Air Force policymakers would need to identify the evidence-based simulation technologies for investment or spread investment across a variety of options, with the risk that relatively low investment in each option would not substantially improve simulation technology or access. Perhaps most important, the level of skill and readiness gained through simulation is likely lower than that gained through direct patient care despite recent advances in simulation technology. Overall, expanding access to evidence-based simulation technologies for a large population of personnel who need to "fight soon" could complement other readiness activities that involve care for real patients.

Practice Activities

Readiness activities in the practice category include multiple options for placing medical personnel in settings that serve patients with more intensive needs than the typical MTF. These activities include expanding trauma care at MTFs; placing medical personnel at civilian Level 1 trauma centers or VAMCs on a full-time or part-time basis; employing medical personnel as instructors and mentors (i.e., a cadre) at C-STARS sites or VAMCs; and promoting ODE with a trauma and critical care focus.

---

[22] Jodi Martinez, "C-STARS Sets New DoD Training Standard with New Simulator," U. S. Air Force, March 8, 2017; Nelson, 2018; Alia-Novobilski, 2018.

[23] Adam Dougherty, "SimX Receives New U.S. Air Force Contracts to Advance VR Training Programs, Explore Space Warfighter Readiness," SimX, May 14, 2021.

[24] Laura L. Wiggins, Janice Sarasnick, and Nathan G. Siemens, "Using Simulation to Train Medical Units for Deployment," *Military Medicine*, Vol. 185, Nos. 3–4, March 2, 2020.

Expanding Trauma Care at MTFs

Many Air Force medical personnel, across all medical specialties, provide care at MTFs as part of their primary duty assignments. While much of this care is routine, preventive, or delivered in outpatient settings, some of the care provided at MTFs is more intensive or complex and is therefore more relevant to readiness. Efforts directed at increasing trauma care, and other advanced procedures and critical care at MTFs, in particular, would provide more opportunities for Air Force medical personnel to meet readiness requirements as part of their existing assignments.

In recent decades, however, the number of trauma patients seen at Air Force MTFs has fallen, due at least in part to a drop in the number of Air Force MTFs and closure of many inpatient facilities.[25] Nevertheless, a small number of existing Air Force MTFs have sought to increase the number of trauma patients they see. The most notable example is the Mike O'Callaghan Military Medical Center at Nellis Air Force Base, Nevada, which is seeking a Level 3 trauma center designation.[26] Providers at other facilities, including Wright-Patterson Air Force Base, have also sought to increase trauma care at MTFs in some instances on an ad hoc basis.[27] Efforts to increase trauma care at other services' MTFs, such as at Brooke Army Medical Center (a Level 1 trauma center) or Naval Medical Center Camp Lejeune (a Level 3 trauma center), can also provide opportunities for Air Force medical personnel assigned to those facilities to gain trauma experience.[28]

Increasing the number of trauma patients seen at an MTF, particularly through its designation as a trauma center and arranging to admit patients from emergency medical services, requires careful coordination with the DHA, local government, medical transport providers, and nearby civilian hospitals. The most promising locations for such efforts may be those that feature an existing Air Force MTF with inpatient facilities, a growing and medically underserved civilian population, a growing number of trauma patients in the region, and receptive local government officials.[29] As part of these arrangements, even MTFs that already provide inpatient services would likely need to increase specialized staffing, resources, and facilities available for trauma

---

[25] John C. Graser, Daniel Blum, Kevin Brancato, James J. Burks, Edward W. Chan, Nancy Nicosia, Michael J. Neumann, Hans V. Ritschard, and Benjamin F. Mundell, *The Economics of Air Force Medical Service Readiness*, RAND Corporation, TR-859-AF, 2010, p. xiv; MHS, *Military Health System Modernization Study Team Report*, Office of the Under Secretary of Defense for Personnel and Readiness, May 29, 2015, p. 11.

[26] Dwane Young, "99th MDG Seeks Trauma Accreditation," Defense Visual Information Distribution Service, July 31, 2020.

[27] Former Air Force Medical Group commander, interview with the authors, March 31, 2021.

[28] Elaine Sanchez, "BAMC Takes On Additional Trauma Patients," U. S. Army, January 7, 2021; Naval Medical Center Camp Lejeune, "Trauma Center," webpage, undated; DoD, *Restructuring and Realignment of Military Medical Treatment Facilities: Report to the Congressional Defense Committees*, Office of the Under Secretary of Defense for Personnel and Readiness, February 19, 2020, p. 11.

[29] Former medical group commander, interview with the authors, July 16, 2021.

care.[30] Obtaining certification as a Level 1, 2, or 3 trauma center from the American College of Surgeons is a labor-intensive and costly process, though there are examples of new trauma centers that have become profitable through billing for services to trauma patients.[31] However, for MTFs, billing civilians and civilian insurance programs for care can pose challenges because this is not a central function of most MTFs.[32]

Establishing a Temporary Duty Within-Skill Exchange Program

Under this option, a medical professional from a low-volume MTF would "trade places" with a medical professional from a high-volume MTF for a month. The exchange would elevate the patient care experience and readiness of the individual from the low-volume MTF; the individual from the high-volume MTF could be selected for his or her capacity to help train and mentor personnel at the low-volume MTF, conferring benefits on the host site. This activity would be most appropriate for personnel who do not have readily available access to trauma experience but could benefit from critical care experience, such as surgeons, nonsurgeon physicians, and nurses. Implementation of such an exchange program would depend on availability of staff to coordinate the exchange, as well as the availability of a person at the high-volume site to serve as a trainer and mentor.

An exchange program would obviate the cost of backfilling positions that are associated with most readiness activities in the practice category (e.g., placing medical personnel from an MTF at a civilian Level 1 trauma center or VAMC). However, it would entail TDY costs for two people. This type of program would also disrupt continuity of patient care at both sites and result in some loss of productivity at the beginning and end of the placement as personnel adjust to a new setting and then return to their original assignments.

Embedding at a Civilian Level 1 Trauma Center

Air Force medical personnel needing the highest level of trauma readiness may be embedded full-time at civilian Level 1 trauma centers under a Training Affiliation Agreement (TAA) between the MTF and the civilian facility. TAAs are subject to legal review, as well as approval by the Office of the Air Force Surgeon General. To be approved, TAAs must provide a "clear benefit" to the Air Force in terms of improving medical personnel's clinical proficiency. In return, the civilian facility benefits from Air Force clinicians providing care for their patients and billing for their services without having to pay the clinicians' salaries, which are covered by the Air

---

[30] American College of Surgeons, Committee on Trauma, *Resources for Optimal Care of the Injured Patient*, 2014.

[31] Megan Masserly and Jackie Valley, "Heated Topic in Health Care: Does Las Vegas Have Enough Trauma Centers?" *Las Vegas Sun*, April 7, 2016.

[32] Jaie Avila, "Legislation Would Allow BAMC to Waive Big, Surprise Bills for Some Patients," News 4 San Antonio, December 18, 2020.

Force.[33] This arrangement is relatively common, with over 1,000 TAAs active in 2017, though most TAAs involve part-time rather than full-time work in civilian facilities.[34]

Under a TAA, Air Force medical personnel are primarily expected to provide direct patient care to civilian trauma patients. Secondary responsibilities may include teaching or mentoring others and supervising trainees. An existing example of embedded Air Force medical personnel is the Air Force Special Operations Command's Special Operations Surgical Teams at the University of Alabama at Birmingham.[35] These highly trained individuals are expected to function at the highest level during in-theater trauma resuscitations.

Since all Air Force medical personnel need to be ready to care for critically ill trauma patients when active conflict occurs, all AFSCs should be eligible to be embedded at a Level 1 trauma center. In practice, however, civilian trauma centers are more receptive to personnel in medical specialties that are in higher demand and have more easily transferred medical credentials, such as surgeons. Embedding personnel at civilian Level 1 trauma centers is likely to be most beneficial to personnel who need to function at the highest level when conflict occurs—that is, surgeons (general surgeons, trauma surgeons, and orthopedic surgeons), emergency physicians, anesthesiologists, critical care nurses, emergency nurses, operating room and surgical nurses, cardiopulmonary laboratory staff, and surgical service staff. Embedding a team of medical personnel would potentially offer the best readiness at the team level, since these individuals would have already fostered trust through shared experiences and be familiar with each team member's strengths and limitations.

Being embedded at a civilian Level 1 trauma center enables routine exposure to patients requiring trauma resuscitation, which is likely the best activity for generating readiness in CONUS. Personnel participating in this activity are then ready to be assigned to PACAF or to be deployed to PACAF as required.

The CMRPs emphasize the importance of both knowledge and procedural performance for clinical currency and readiness; routine resuscitation of patients experiencing penetrating and blunt trauma is likely to lead embedded personnel to excel in both knowledge and performance. However, because this readiness building activity is relatively costly for the workforce (it requires the "loss" of one FTE from an MTF to a civilian trauma center), it is currently uncommon.

If the Air Force were to invest in this option and gradually build toward even 5 percent of critical medical personnel embedded in civilian trauma centers, that would entail participation

---

[33] Air Force Manual 41-108, *Training Affiliation Agreement Program*, Department of the Air Force, August 21, 2019.

[34] Mark Ediger, "Air Force Medical Service: Focus Areas in Action," Headquarters U.S. Air Force, briefing, February 9, 2017, p. 8.

[35] Daniel B. Cox, "Managing a Mature Military-Civilian Partnership: Civilian Perspective," UAB School of Medicine, briefing, undated.

from approximately 500 personnel (i.e., 500 FTEs). If 25 personnel were embedded at each civilian Level 1 trauma center, the Air Force would require a total of 20 such sites; achieving this number would require substantial costs, time, and logistical efforts to create the necessary TAAs. Additionally, the disadvantage of embedding Air Force medical personnel at a civilian facility is the possible erosion of military acculturation over time in comparison with practice at an MTF. Furthermore, this option (and all options that remove uniformed personnel from MTFs) will require hiring civilian or contractor replacement staff, which might present challenges.

Doubling the Size of the C-STARS Cadres

C-STARS students deliver care to civilian patients under the supervision of C-STARS instructors, who are also known as cadre members, and receive a mix of classroom instruction and simulation training. C-STARS cadre members, in addition to supervising these students, also provide direct patient care and build capacity to teach trauma care skills.

This activity would double the number of cadre members without increasing the number of students. As a result, there would be more than one cadre member from each AFSC at each C-STARS site, minimizing disruption to training and patient care in case of a large deployment that drew from C-STARS cadres. The activity would halve the teaching workload but allow for twice as many deployments. When deployed, cadre members would function as experts on trauma care (i.e., "trauma czars") in the deployed setting and leverage their teaching experience to enhance the trauma care skills of others. Thus, this activity would enhance the readiness of cadre members and those around them. In a major national defense emergency, C-STARS could be suspended, and the entire cadre of expert trauma care providers and teachers could be made available for deployment.

This activity would have several advantages and challenges. It would double the number of C-STARS cadre members from 65 to 130; therefore, the manpower costs would double, and there would be additional associated overhead costs for amending agreements.[36] The activity would produce a small corps of deployment-ready medical personnel with a high degree of trauma expertise. Infrastructure for C-STARS already exists, and civilian hospitals that host C-STARS sites would benefit from the availability of more medical professionals to provide civilian care. However, an expansion of cadres might provoke opposition from physician groups, nurses' unions, or other entities that could perceive cadre members as taking away civilian jobs.

Encouraging Intermittent Practice at Civilian Level 1 Trauma Centers

Air Force medical personnel assigned to an MTF can work at a trauma center or other civilian medical facility on a part-time basis in addition to their primary duty assignment under a TAA. Medical personnel in high-demand career fields and who possess credentials that easily transfer

---

[36] The existing 65 cadre members include a recent average of 24 members at C-STARS Baltimore, 18 at C-STARS St. Louis, and 23 at C-STARS Cincinnati from 2018 to 2020.

to civilian medical facilities are most likely to find part-time work at a civilian trauma center. These personnel include trauma surgeons, orthopedic surgeons, anesthesiologists, emergency services physicians, and critical care nurses. Aerospace medical technicians and enlisted personnel in other career fields are less able to take advantage of opportunities to work in a civilian trauma center, though they may be able to gain experience from part-time work under TAAs with other civilian medical facilities or prehospital medical transportation services.[37]

Most part-time work at civilian trauma centers involves Air Force medical personnel working individually alongside their civilian counterparts rather than providing care as part of a team of military clinicians. Gaining experience in trauma care is central to Air Force medical personnel readiness and is explicitly required by many career field CMRPs. Given that the vast majority of peacetime trauma care is provided at civilian facilities, part-time work in these facilities is a relatively common way to fulfill these requirements, at least for the more specialized medical officer career fields.[38]

The expense associated with this activity is a manpower cost equal to the time spent away from the MTF for each individual, which is often between one-tenth and one-third FTE. A limited number of individuals might require TDY coverage for travel to institutions that are not located near a primary MTF. Additionally, small overhead costs are necessary to create and maintain TAAs to facilitate intermittent practice agreements.

Embedding at a Veterans Affairs Medical Center

Air Force medical personnel from certain specialties needing to enhance knowledge and performance in critical care could be embedded at VA facilities that have a large volume of critically ill patients. Under this arrangement, a nearby affiliated MTF would have oversight over Air Force medical personnel, but the personnel would care for patients full-time at the VAMC. To our knowledge, this arrangement is rarely used today; and it would require a memorandum of understanding (MOU) between the MTF, the VAMC, and, in some cases, medical schools to facilitate this readiness option.[39]

We envision that physician critical care specialists, such as anesthesiologists, pulmonologists, and critical care nurses, could benefit from this arrangement if they would otherwise be practicing at an MTF. The volume of critically ill patients at MTFs tends to be low because TRICARE

---

[37] Current medical group commander, interview with the authors, May 6, 2021; former medical group commander, interview with the authors, July 16, 2021; Deputy Group Commander Chief Nurse, undated, p. 24; American College of Surgeons, *The Blue Book: Military-Civilian Partnerships for Trauma Training, Sustainment, and Readiness*, 2020, pp. 6–7.

[38] Ediger, 2017, p. 8.

[39] According to one presentation, there were only 54 DoD-VA MOUs for medical personnel in 2017; Ediger, 2017, p. 8.

beneficiaries tend to be young and healthy.[40] In contrast, more than half of VA beneficiaries are 65 or older, and they have high rates of medical and mental health comorbidities that place them at risk for critical illness.[41] To meet this critical care need, 117 of 139 VAMCs (84 percent) had medical intensive care units in 2012, which provide care for 30,000 patients nationwide annually.[42]

For Air Force medical personnel who require proficiency and readiness related to high-acuity care, being embedded at a VAMC would likely allow them to gain experience caring for medically complex patients, including through the performance of procedures such as central line placement and endotracheal intubations. This readiness-generating activity would not, however, increase exposure to trauma patients requiring resuscitation because VAMCs do not receive trauma patients by ambulance. The majority of exposure to trauma patients at VAMCs would be care for patients with severe brain and spinal cord injuries who were resuscitated elsewhere and then transferred to a VAMC for longer-term rehabilitation.[43]

Other nonphysician Air Force medical personnel requiring experience in operating rooms could also benefit from being embedded at a VAMC. For example, operating room nurses, surgical technologists, and cardiopulmonary laboratory personnel could gain experience in operating rooms that might not always be available in an MTF. Nurses might face barriers in obtaining positions as embedded personnel at VAMCs due to opposition from nursing unions. IDMTs might also face barriers to readiness-generating activities at VAs, due to misalignment between their skills in the military and allowable roles in domestic medical facilities.

Implementation of this activity might depend on the ability of the VA to reimburse the Air Force for services provided by Air Force medical personnel at VAMCs. Federal law provides for sharing of health care resources between DoD and the VA for the mutual benefit of the two departments, and they "have an organizational structure in place to plan and carry out a variety of joint projects and collaboration efforts."[44] The two departments have a variety of sharing agreements in place covering clinical care, graduate medical education, and nonmedical services.

---

[40] Health.mil, "Patient Care Numbers for the Miliary Health System," webpage, undated-a; Health.mil, "Patients by TRICARE Plan," webpage, undated-b.

[41] RAND Corporation, *Assessment A (Demographics)*, September 1, 2015; Matthew S. Goldberg, "Comparing the Costs of the Veterans' Health Care System with Private-Sector Costs," testimony before the Subcommittee on Health, Committee on Veterans' Affairs, U.S. House of Representatives, Congressional Budget Office, January 28, 2015.

[42] VA, Veterans Health Administration, *2012 VHA Facility Quality and Safety* Report, September 2012; Lena M. Chen, Marta Render, Anne Sales, Edward H. Kennedy, Wyndy Wiitala, and Timothy P. Hofer, "Intensive Care Unit Admitting Patterns in the Veterans Affairs Health Care System," *Archives of Internal Medicine*, Vol. 172, No. 16, September 2012.

[43] VHA Interagency Health Affairs, "DoD/VA Sharing Agreements," U.S. Department of Veterans Affairs and U.S. Department of Defense, briefing, undated.

[44] VHA Interagency Health Affairs, undated; U.S. Government Accountability Office, *VA and DoD Health Care: Department-Level Actions Needed to Assess Collaboration Performance, Address Barriers, and Identify Opportunities*, GAO-12-992, September 2012.

While it is unclear whether the VA could reimburse DoD for time spent by Air Force personnel to provide care at VAMCs under existing agreements, the history and organizational structure for cooperation between the two departments could facilitate this readiness-generating activity. Moreover, the VA might benefit from this activity, as well as the other activities that would embed Air Force medical personnel at VAMCs either full- or part-time. An informant reported that many VA hospitals have difficulty hiring providers due to compensation constraints within the federal government's General Schedule classification and pay system for civilian employees.[45] As a result, the VA may be willing to work with the Air Force to help fill gaps.

In addition to performing direct patient care, Air Force medical personnel embedded at VAMCs could also play a role in teaching and mentoring other Air Force medical personnel who rotate part-time through a VAMC. We have learned from key informants that, without having embedded personnel or cadres, experiences for part-time Air Force personnel may be inadequate at enhancing readiness because full-time non-MHS personnel may not allow rotators to perform procedures or become involved in direct patient care.[46]

If the Air Force were to invest in this option and gradually build toward 5 percent of critical care specialists embedded in VAMCs,[47] this would amount to approximately 21 personnel (i.e., 21 FTEs). If five personnel were embedded at each embedding site, the Air Force would require a total of five sites; achieving this number would require moderate costs, time, and logistical efforts to create the necessary MOUs. Additionally, once embedding has been achieved, the Air Force could consider embedding additional nurses without critical care backgrounds at VAMC sites to help them achieve the critical care hours necessary to gain certification from the American Association of Critical Care Nurses.[48]

Establishing Veterans Affairs Medical Center Cadres

Establishing VAMC cadres would mirror the option of embedding Air Force medical personnel at VAMCs, with the modification that cadre members would allocate a substantial portion of their time at the VAMC to teaching and mentoring other Air Force personnel who rotate through the facility. Thus, this option would help maintain readiness for cadre members and support readiness of other Air Force personnel. A cadre member could teach a structured course or curriculum or simply play the role of a liaison who mentors and supports intermittent Air Force personnel. At maximum, 20 cadre members would be embedded at each VAMC if their role included teaching a structured curriculum; this is roughly the same size as the existing cadre at each of the C-STARS trauma programs. Fewer cadre members could be embedded if

---

[45] Senior leader, AFMS, interview with the authors, June 10, 2021.

[46] Former medical group commander, interview with the authors, July 16, 2021.

[47] Here we define critical care specialists as those in the following AFSCs: Anesthesiologist, 45AX; Internist, Pulmonary Diseases, 44MXG; and Clinical Nurse, Critical Care, 46NXE.

[48] American Association of Critical-Care Nurses, "Board Certification," webpage, undated.

their role was restricted to general overseeing and mentoring. This option would be focused on anesthesiologists, pulmonologists, and critical care nurses, with the possibility of extending to other specialties. It would have similar advantages and challenges to embedding Air Force personnel at a VAMC but with the addition of teaching responsibilities.

Expanding Opportunities for Intermittent Practice at Veterans Affairs Medical Centers

This activity would function similarly to embedding Air Force medical personnel at VAMCs, but it would involve a primary assignment to an MTF and only a part-time role at the VAMC. Duties at the VAMC would include direct patient care and could also include teaching. As we have noted, the VA population is older than the MTF population on average, with higher rates of medical and mental health comorbidities. As a result, providing care for this population would help Air Force medical personnel maintain skills in critical care.

As with the activity of embedding Air Force personnel at VAMCs, this activity would be most appropriate for anesthesiologists, pulmonologists, and critical care nurses. If piloting with those specialists proved to be successful at increasing exposure to critical care, other personnel could also potentially benefit such as physician assistants, cardiopulmonary laboratory personnel, surgical service personnel, and some specialties within Aerospace Medical Service. Clinical nurses, operating room nurses, and advance practice registered nurses might also benefit, though collective bargaining agreements might present a barrier to entry.[49] Because VAMCs do not receive trauma patients by ambulance, this option would not be appropriate for personnel who need to maintain trauma skills, such as emergency services physicians and the independent duty medical technician specialty within Aerospace Medical Service.

This activity would have several potential advantages and challenges. While it may contribute less to readiness than embedding medical personnel at a VAMC full-time, it could offer a flexible option for critical care personnel who do not need to "fight tonight" but who need to "fight soon."

In addition to enhancing critical care readiness, this option could benefit MTFs by spreading critical care skills from VAMC facilities to MTFs via Air Force personnel who divide their time between sites. However, it could also disrupt continuity of care for MTF patients. There are 172 VAMCs and 1,069 outpatient sites across the United States,[50] providing a wide variety of options for Air Force medical personnel who would divide their time between an MTF and a VAMC, but take-up of the opportunity to work part-time at a VAMC might be limited if part-time ODE provides better pay.

---

[49] Air Force representative from the University of Alabama at Birmingham, interview with the authors, May 11, 2021.

[50] Veterans Navigator, "Veterans Health Administration: Where Do I Get the Care I Need?" webpage, last updated May 3, 2021.

An MTF would oversee the Air Force personnel under a TAA between the MTF and the VAMC, but Air Force personnel would allocate only one-tenth to one-third of an FTE to duties at the VAMC. For example, if an Air Force medical professional allocated one-fifth of an FTE at a VAMC, that FTE would spend 52 workdays, or 416 hours, at the facility per year.

Overall, this activity could be a useful complement to other activities that are more appropriate for Air Force medical personnel who provide emergency care and for personnel who provide nonemergency critical care and need to be ready to "fight tonight" by providing a flexible option for nonemergency personnel who need to be ready to "fight soon."

Emphasizing Off-Duty Employment with a Trauma or Critical Care Focus

In some cases, Air Force medical personnel may be able to pursue ODE in trauma or high-acuity care at a civilian hospital. In many ways, this option resembles assigning personnel part-time to a civilian trauma center or VAMC (discussed earlier in this chapter), as the actual work performed—number of hours, types of procedures, integration with civilian colleagues, and others—could be similar. Yet unlike that or any of the other activities, finding and performing ODE requires a greater degree of individual initiative, as well as working additional hours on top of one's existing full-time assignment duties. However, it also comes with additional compensation at civilian pay scales, which can be especially substantial for the more specialized and highly credentialed medical specialties.

Pursuing ODE requires an Air Force medical professional to obtain permission from his or her commander and to apply to and be hired by a civilian medical facility.[51] Obtaining permission depends greatly on whether an MTF commander supports or discourages ODE.[52] Applying to and being hired by a civilian medical facility also depends on a number of factors, including local demand for part-time medical professionals, availability of part-time job openings compatible with active-duty responsibilities, and possession of the medical credentials and clinical experience expected for competitive candidates. Surgeons, anesthesiologists, critical care nurses, and other highly credentialed and in-demand medical specialties tend to be those for whom ODE is often a possibility.[53]

Some AFMS officers expressed concern that ODE could have negative impacts on Air Force medical providers' performance of their military duties, have negative impacts on their retention, and pose ethical challenges given the monetary incentives involved.[54] While Air Force medical providers are required by Air Force Instruction 44-102 to apply for annual leave to cover ODE

---

[51] Air Force Instruction 44-102, *Medical Care Management*, Department of the Air Force, March 17, 2015.

[52] One recent study found that, at least in the Army, "some surgeons felt that ODE was unsupported by their MTF commander and by the Army at large and were consequently discouraged from utilizing this avenue"; Chan, Krull, Ahluwalia, Broyles, Waxman, Gurvey, Colthirst, Schimmels, and Marinos, 2020, p. 33.

[53] Former medical group commander, interview with the authors, July 16, 2021.

[54] PACAF Surgeon General's staff, discussions with the authors, September 21, 2021.

that would occur during duty hours, AFMS stakeholders stated that a pilot program is allowing for exceptions to this rule in some cases.[55] The direct cost of this activity is currently minimal, as it only requires permission from an MTF commander and no financial investment by the Air Force.

Chapter Summary

The characteristics of the training and practice readiness activities presented in this chapter vary widely and are summarized in Table 3.2. The table represents an initial attempt to characterize the activities; future research could investigate each and determine the effectiveness for a given AFSC, type of assignment, or location. Training activities are perhaps the easiest options to increase currency because they can be focused directly on trauma and high-acuity care, have low manpower costs and time commitment, and require little coordination outside the Air Force. Some options, such as advanced simulation training, would require additional investment to expand opportunities for participation.

A wide variety of readiness building activities in the practice category can also be used to improve clinical currency and medical readiness. They vary in cost, time commitment required, ease of implementation (depending on location of personnel), and other factors. For example, opportunities to focus on trauma full-time can be effective at building high levels of readiness to provide wartime care, though these activities also entail higher manpower costs. The activities identified during our research offer a robust set of options that can be evaluated for use across the AFMS.

In Chapter 5 we present a prototype method by which the PACAF Surgeon General or the AFMS as a whole can systematically review the activities in Table 3.2 for different situations, including the requirements of different AFSCs.

---

[55] PACAF Surgeon General's staff, discussions with the authors, September 21, 2021; Air Force Instruction 44-102, 2015, section 2.27.4.8.

Table 3.2. Characteristics of Training and Practice Readiness Building Activities

Activity	Mode	Patient Type	Required Coordination Outside the AFMS	Estimated Cost to the Air Force[a]		Participant Time Commitment	Familiarity of the AFMS with Activity	Potential Time to Maturation
				Additive Manpower	Additive Resources			
Training								
Mandating training at C-STARS before or during PACAF assignment	Classroom, simulation, direct patient care	Trauma	None	Low	Low	2 weeks	High	Short (0–2 years)
Developing a traveling trauma course	Classroom, simulation	Trauma	None	Low	Medium	2–5 days	Low	Medium (2–4 years)
Investing in simulation training	Simulation	Trauma	New and expanded contracts with simulation providers	Low	Medium to high	N/A	Medium	Long (4–10 years)
Practice								
Expanding trauma care at MTFs	Direct patient care	Trauma	Coordination required with DHA, as well as local civilian community, health providers, and government	Medium	High	Full-time	Medium	Long (4–10 years)
Establishing a TDY within-skill exchange program	Direct patient care	Varies with location; goal is trauma and/or high acuity	None	Low	Low	4–8 weeks	Low	Medium (2–4 years)
Embedding at a civilian Level 1 trauma center	Direct patient care	Trauma	New and expanded TAAs with civilian trauma centers	High	Low	Full-time	Medium	Medium (2–4 years)
Doubling the size of the	Teaching, direct patient care	Trauma	Expanded TAAs with civilian trauma centers hosting C-STARS	High	Low	Full-time	High	Medium (2–4 years)

Activity	Mode	Patient Type	Required Coordination Outside the AFMS	Estimated Cost to the Air Force[a]		Participant Time Commitment	Familiarity of the AFMS with Activity	Potential Time to Maturation
				Additive Manpower	Additive Resources			
C-STARS cadres								
Encouraging intermittent practice at civilian Level 1 trauma center	Direct patient care	Trauma	New and expanded TAAs with civilian trauma centers	Medium	Low	Part-time	High	Short (0–2 years)
Embedding at a VAMC	Direct patient care	High-acuity nontrauma	New and expanded MOUs with VA	High	Low	Full-time	Low	Medium (2–4 years)
Establishing VAMC cadres	Teaching, direct patient care	High-acuity nontrauma	New and expanded MOUs with VA	High	Low	Full-time	Low	Medium (2–4 years)
Expanding opportunities for intermittent practice at VAMCs	Direct patient care	High-acuity nontrauma	New and expanded MOUs with VA	Medium	Low	Part-time	Medium	Short (0–2 years)
Emphasizing ODE with a critical care focus	Direct patient care	Varies with location; goal is trauma and/or high acuity	None	Low	Low	Part-time	Medium	Short (0–2 years)

[a] Cost categories are relative to the options we present in the table.

Chapter 4. Readiness Building: Assignment Policies

Air Force medical personnel are moved from assignment to assignment in the same way that those in other career fields are. Assignments are governed by Air Force Instruction 36-2110 and depend on Air Force needs, individual preferences, individual readiness and career development, and other factors. Air Force Instruction 36-2110 also prescribes tour lengths, which vary based on location, accompanied status, and mission requirements.[1]

The project sponsor and other subject-matter experts have suggested that adjusting assignment policies for medical AFSCs could mitigate the potential decline of knowledge and skill proficiency and readiness, especially in PACAF. This could be the case, for example, if individuals passed through high-volume locations before being assigned to PACAF to ensure that they had high proficiency when they arrived in-theater, or by limiting the duration of assignments at low-volume locations in PACAF to reduce time for skill decay.

This chapter continues our discussion of readiness building activities by exploring policies linked to assignments. We first present a brief description of three assignment policies that could improve the proficiency and readiness of medical personnel. The outcomes for these policies vary by AFSC and shredout and are dependent on the number and type of positions at locations throughout the AFMS. Therefore, to understand the effects of these assignment policies on proficiency by AFSC, we developed an analytic framework to simulate these effects.

Assignment Policies

We evaluated three potential changes to assignment policy: reducing tour lengths at low-volume WestPac locations, sequencing assignments to maintain or improve proficiency, and using nonmilitary personnel to fill positions at CONUS medical facilities with low patient volumes.

Reducing Tour Lengths at Low-Volume Western Pacific Locations

Assignment lengths vary across WestPac locations from 12 to 36 months, with extensions for longer tours allowed in some circumstances.[2] During discussions with the PACAF Surgeon General's staff, previous medical group commanders at WestPac locations, and consultants, it was suggested numerous times that keeping people at remote PACAF locations where skills may atrophy due to low patient volume was problematic. They agreed that limiting time at these low-

[1] Air Force Instruction 36-2110, *Total Force Assignments*, Department of the Air Force, November 15, 2021.

[2] Tour lengths for some locations and AFSCs in WestPac have already been shortened to 24 months.

volume locations and allowing medical personnel to move to locations where their proficiency could be maintained or improved could be beneficial.

To examine the broad potential effect of this policy option, we conducted an initial analysis simulating the effect of reducing WestPac assignments to 12 months for all critical medical specialties. In the future, a more detailed analysis taking into account specific location characteristics and duty requirements for different AFSCs could simulate the effects of assignment durations tailored to specific WestPac locations and medical specialties. A more detailed analysis could also determine the estimated added costs for additional permanent change-of-station moves required under this policy.

Sequencing Assignments to Maintain or Improve Proficiency

The AFPC is the organization responsible for assigning personnel to fill positions across the Air Force. Several factors influence these assignment decisions, including, for many of the specialties, recommended career paths as personnel gain experience and rank. For medical AFSCs, specialty consultants are also involved, especially for assigning individuals to leadership positions or those that require special skills or training. Individual medical professionals also have an opportunity to express preferences regarding their assignments.

Assignments at some locations can increase proficiency, while at others proficiency may decline depending on the volume and opportunity to practice required skills. Discussions with the project sponsor, other AFMS subject-matter experts, and representatives from the AFPC did not reveal whether assignment decisions are being made with a goal of maintaining or increasing proficiency from an enterprise level. A policy that did consider proficiency might make it a priority to send an individual assigned to a low-volume, noncritical care location to a high-volume critical care location for their following assignment to build back proficiency.

For our analysis, we divided all assignment locations into two tiers based on their likely potential to either increase or decrease personnel medical proficiency due to having a relatively higher or lower patient volume. We categorized locations with an inpatient hospital, a military medical training facility such as C-STARS or Las Vegas SMART, or a civilian trauma center—all of which tend to feature higher patient volumes and complexity of care—as Tier 1. All other locations were categorized as Tier 2 (including WestPac MTFs). (For a list of locations, see Table A.1.) This is a simplifying assumption; certain individuals at a Tier 1 location may nonetheless experience a lower-than-expected case load due to the responsibilities of their position, while individuals at a Tier 2 location may be assigned duties that enhance their proficiency. Future analysis efforts could improve the fidelity with which positions are judged to increase or decrease proficiency by considering such factors as acuity, complexity, staffing and bed days.

Historically, individuals assigned to WestPac have come from a mixture of Tier 1 and Tier 2 locations. For the initial analysis tested in this research, however, we prioritize assignments to WestPac from Tier 1 locations to ensure that individuals have high proficiency and readiness should their skills be needed. This policy may also prevent an individual's proficiency from declining to unacceptable levels from which it would be difficult to recover while assigned to a WestPac location.

Using the Military Workforce at High-Volume, and Nonmilitary Personnel at Low-Volume, CONUS Locations

The civilian and contractor workforce is an "open system"; and personnel with varying specialties, levels of expertise, and experience can be hired as required. In contrast, the military workforce is generally a "closed system," with personnel entering at junior, inexperienced levels and gaining experience, responsibilities, and rank all while serving in the Air Force.[3] Notably, initial treatment of wartime casualties will largely be provided by uniformed medical personnel. Taking these workforce characteristics into consideration, an enterprise-level approach might retain positions where trauma and critical care skills are practiced most for military medical providers. In doing so, civilian and contract workers would be assigned to less-complex peacetime medical care. At least some of these civilian and contract workers will be additive to the existing manpower in critical medical specialties, so there are likely costs associated with employing these workers.

Through our review of the literature and in discussions with subject-matter experts, we observed that decisions to fill positions with civilians and contracted personnel are often made at the local level. Consequently, civilians and contractors are present in positions in both Tier 1 and Tier 2 locations.

To assess the impact of this policy on the proficiency of military medical personnel, we simulated increasing the manning at Tier 1 locations by up to 25 percent (up to a maximum of 110 percent of authorizations).[4] This increase is offset by a proportional reduction in manning at CONUS Tier 2 locations. By placing more military individuals at Tier 1 locations, we hypothesize that proficiency will increase across the AFMS, as well as in WestPac specifically, as individuals will have higher proficiency on average when they arrive.[5]

Simulating Assignment Policies

To assess the effect of assignment policy changes on the proficiency levels of medical personnel, we developed an analytic framework that contains modeling and simulation components, as Figure 4.1 illustrates. In the assignment model, historical personnel data are used to obtain

---

[3] In some AFSCs (e.g., in the nurse corps), members do enter at grades from second lieutenant to major with as much as 20 years of civilian experience prior to entering.

[4] A potential drawback is that this could reduce cases per provider at Tier 1 locations, reducing some of the benefit.

[5] This assumes that the demand for the services of an AFSC at a particular Tier 1 location is sufficiently high to meet the experiential needs of up to 25 percent more medical professionals.

statistics on the probability that an individual will separate, be reassigned at a point in time, and, if reassigned, move from location A to location B. The proficiency of an individual is also modeled as a function of whether an MTF is considered a Tier 1 or Tier 2 location. These statistical models are then used to simulate the assignments of individuals in the future periods while observing the changes in proficiency. When combined with analyst-specified changes to the statistical models, it is possible to simulate the impact of assignment policies on proficiency

Figure 4.1. The Modeling and Simulation Methodology

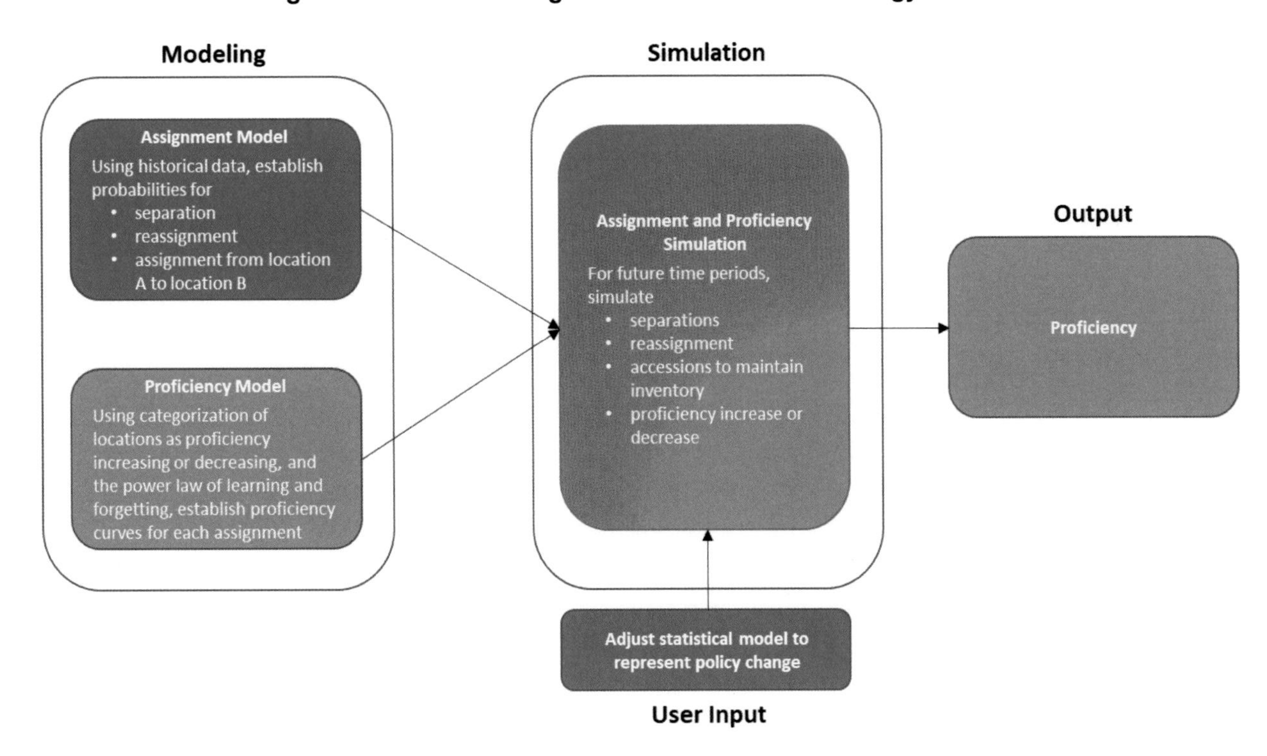

and observe the resulting manning, tour lengths, and assignment sequences. Additional information on this framework is provided in Appendix A.

Modeling and Simulating the Assignment System

We created a statistical model that emulates the dynamics of the assignment system over the previous 11 years and can be used to forecast assignment dynamics and readiness over an indefinite number of future years.[6] This effort involved using historical data from 2010 to 2020 to estimate four sets of probabilities and probability distributions for each critical medical AFSC:

1. **Initial assignment location:** the distribution of initial assignments across locations. These values influence where individuals begin their careers.

---

[6] We gathered monthly officer and enlisted personnel extracts from the Military Personnel Data System from calendar year (CY) 2010 through CY 2020. We used multiple years' worth of data to more reliably estimate probabilistic inputs to the simulation framework. All reported simulations correspond to a 20-year future time horizon.

2. **Assignment sequence:** the probability that an individual at location A will next be assigned to location B, for all possible pairs of locations A and B. These values influence assignment sequences.
3. **Assignment probability:** the monthly probability of moving from one assignment to another given current assignment location and time on station (TOS). These values influence tour lengths.
4. **Separation probability:** the monthly probability of separating from the Air Force for a given location, TOS, and YOS. These values influence career lengths.

We used the statistical model to simulate future year effects of changes to assignment policies. We seeded the simulation with the current inventory (i.e., individuals by location, TOS, and YOS), and we held the size of the inventory constant by setting accessions to maintain career field strength observed during the year prior to the simulation.[7]

Each simulation cycle consisted of five events that occurred on a monthly basis: (1) computing monthly separations; (2) computing monthly assignments; (3) reassigning individuals to maintain manning levels by location and in accord with historical assignment sequences; (4) accessing the number of individuals needed to maintain overall AFSC end strength and with initial assignments based on the historical distribution; and (5) aging the inventory.[8] In actuality, the number of accessions and assignments would not perfectly offset losses from a given location. Yet this simplifying assumption provides a reasonable approximation of the average dynamics across years where the goal is to maintain the size of the force. The simulation produced a complete person-month record that begins from the current inventory and extends 20 years into the future.

Modeling and Simulating Proficiency

In addition to the model of the assignment system discussed previously, which provides a simulation of where people are assigned, a method for modeling the proficiency of individuals as they move through these assignments is also needed. The acquisition and retention of knowledge and skills depends on many factors, two of which are the amount of practice and the elapsed time since practice occurred. During periods of use, proficiency tends to increase according to a power law of learning: initial practice produces large gains, and additional practice produces further gains but at a diminishing rate. Conversely, during periods of disuse, proficiency changes according to a power law of forgetting: initial periods of disuse produce large losses, and additional disuse produces further losses but at a diminishing rate.[9] The power law of learning and the power law of forgetting are extremely general. They have been observed in virtually

---

[7] The current inventory reflects manning at the start of January 2021. Because manning levels have historically fluctuated, target career field strengths in the simulation were set to values recently observed during CY 2020.

[8] The choice to use monthly time steps is a simplification; many of the processes modeled (e.g., accession, separation, and assignment) occur continuously.

[9] Matthew M. Walsh and Marsha Lovett, "The Cognitive Science Approach to Learning and Memory," in Susan Chipman, ed., *The Oxford Handbook of Cognitive Science*, Oxford: Oxford University Press, 2016.

every domain, including education, psychomotor abilities, and performance of complex military and medical tasks.[10]

To simulate the acquisition and retention of clinical proficiency, we made the simplifying assumption that, on average, individuals in critical medical specialties gain proficiency when they are assigned to a location with high clinical volume and that they lose proficiency when they are assigned to a location with low clinical volume. Over the course of an individual's career, this produces an ebb and flow characterized by periods of high proficiency after being assigned to locations with an inpatient hospital, a military medical training facility, or a civilian trauma center (i.e., Tier 1 locations),[11] and periods of lower proficiency after being assigned to low-volume locations (i.e., Tier 2 locations). Appendix A contains a list of labeled locations.

Figure 4.2 shows the simulated proficiency for two hypothetical medical professionals. Both complete an initial 24-month assignment at a Tier 1 location, during which time they build proficiency. Airman Smith is then assigned to a Tier 2 location, and Airman Brown is assigned to another Tier 1 location. Airman Smith loses proficiency during the second assignment, while Airman Brown continues to build proficiency but at a diminishing rate. Finally, Airman Smith is assigned once again to a Tier 1 location, and Airman Brown is assigned to a Tier 2 location for the first time. Airman Smith rebuilds proficiency during the third assignment, while Airman Brown loses proficiency.

---

[10] John R. Anderson and Christian D. Schunn, "Implications of the ACT-R Learning Theory: No Magic Bullets," in Robert Glaser, ed., *Advances in Instructional Psychology*: Vol. 5, *Educational Design and Cognitive Science*, Lawrence Erlbaum Associates, Inc., 2000; Arthur, Bennett, Stanush, and McNelly, 1998; Perez, Skinner, Weyhrauch, Niehaus, Lathan, Schwaitzberg, and Cao, 2013.

[11] An example of a location with a military medical training facility is Brooke Army Medical Center.

Figure 4.2. Simulated Proficiency for Two Individuals over 96 Months

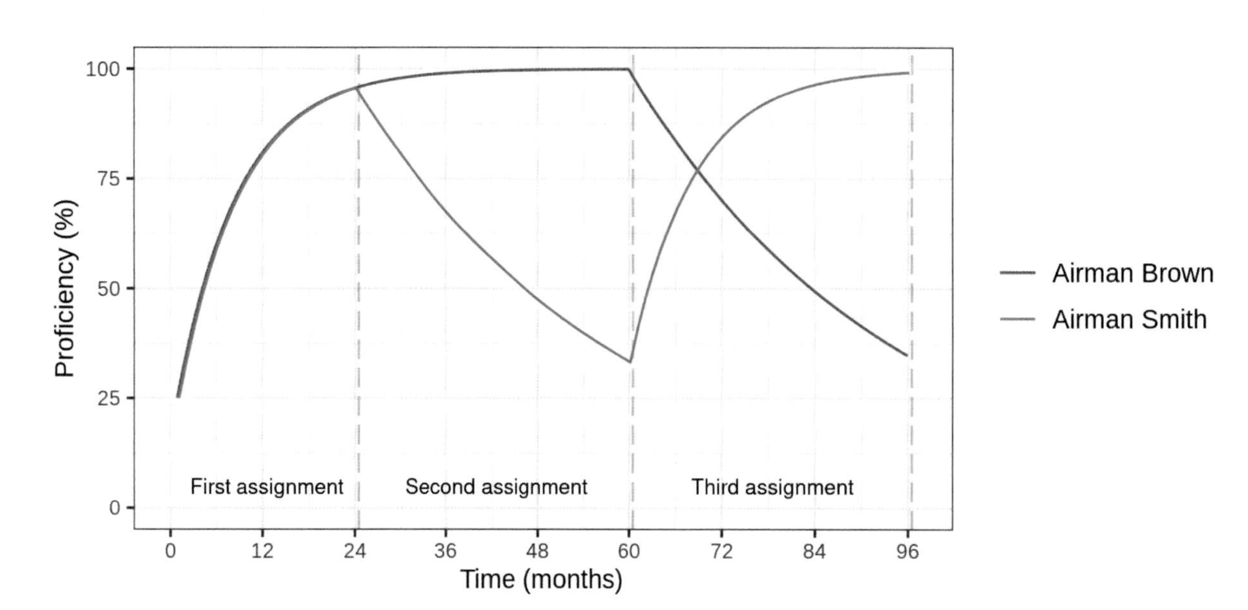

Our cognitive model of skill acquisition and decay applies these dynamics longitudinally to individuals based on the assignment locations, durations, and sequences they experience in the simulation. The output of the cognitive model, a continuous value that increases with time spent at Tier 1 locations and decreases with time spent at Tier 2 locations, can be used to compare the effects of different policy options on the clinical proficiency of individuals during certain key assignments. For example, Airman Smith has higher proficiency than Airman Brown at the end of the third assignment. If one of the two individuals must then fill a vacancy in WestPac, and if the goal is to maximize the proficiency of individuals in WestPac, it would be most beneficial to assign Airman Smith to that region. Additionally, the proficiency curves decrease with time spent at Tier 2 locations. If the goal is to maximize the proficiency of individuals in WestPac, it would also be beneficial to assign Airman Brown to that region for far less than three years.

Modeling and Simulation Framework Assumptions and Outputs

The simulation makes three simplifying assumptions:

1. Skill acquisition and decay follow a power law of learning and a power law of forgetting. Additionally, learning and decay rates are similar for individuals and for different clinical tasks. Although these are reasonable assumptions, more complex models of skill acquisition and retention exist, and some models account for individual and task differences.[12]

---

[12] Tiffany S. Jastrzembski, Matthew M. Walsh, Michael Krusmark, Suzan Kardong-Edgren, Marilyn H. Oermann, Karey Dufour, Teresa Millwater, Kevin Gluck, Glenn Gunzelmann, Jack Harris, and Dimitrios Stefanidis, "Personalizing Training to Acquire and Sustain Competence Through Use of a Cognitive Model," in Dylan D.

2. Each location features either a higher (Tier 1) or a lower (Tier 2) clinical case volume, which determines whether the individuals assigned to that location build or lose proficiency. This assumption does not consider the potential for individuals to augment skills through training programs or part-time work in civilian settings, nor does it consider the different clinical duties of individuals assigned to the same location. Further, it assumes the mobility of individuals between Tier 1 and Tier 2 locations.
3. Changes to assignment sequences and tour lengths will not negatively affect retention and other aspects of the personnel inventory. This assumption does not account for the potentially negative indirect effects of the assignment policy options on career satisfaction and continuation.

Given these assumptions, the simulation outputs can be used to estimate the effectiveness of implementing different combinations of policy options and to determine which are most effective for increasing clinical proficiency for different AFSCs. The absolute proficiency values computed by the simulation (e.g., an average proficiency value of 75 percent for all personnel within a particular AFSC) depend in part on the model specifications and parameters used. To examine the robustness of the proficiency results, we replicated the simulations using a wide range of model parameter values for skill acquisition and decay rates (see Appendix A for details).

The proficiency value returned by the model can be mapped to a variety of performance measures. For example, power laws have been fitted to computer-based evaluations of performance and expert evaluations of performance, efficiency, and clinical outcome measures.[13] To tailor the output of the computational cognitive model to the AFMS in the future, relevant performance outcomes must be identified and measured. The model can then be fitted with this newly collected data and used to better predict specific performance outcomes that are relevant to the AFMS.

The Impact of Assignment Policies

We examined the three assignment policies individually and in combination and compared the results with a baseline where no policy changes were implemented. Thus, for each AFSC we calculate estimates for eight cases:

1. baseline
2. reduced assignment duration at WestPac locations
3. prioritized sequencing for WestPac locations
4. increased manning at Tier 1 locations
5. reduced duration *and* prioritized sequencing

Schmorrow and Cali M. Fidopiastis, eds., *Augmented Cognition: Enhancing Cognition and Behavior in Complex Human Environments*, Springer, 2017; Matthew M. Walsh, Kevin A. Gluck, Glenn Gunzelmann, Tiffany Jastrzembski, and Michael Krusmark, "Evaluating the Theoretic Adequacy and Applied Potential of Computational Models of the Spacing Effect," *Cognitive Science*, Vol. 42, No. S3, 2018.

[13] Carol-Anne E. Moulton, Adam Dubrowski, Helen MacRae, Brent Graham, Ethan Grober, and Richard Reznick, "Teaching Surgical Skills: What Kind of Practice Makes Perfect? A Randomized, Controlled Trial, *Annals of Surgery*, Vol. 244, No. 3, 2006.

6. reduced duration *and* increased Tier 1 manning
7. prioritized sequencing *and* increased Tier 1 manning
8. reduced duration, prioritized sequencing, *and* increased Tier 1 manning.

We simulated the 20 largest critical medical AFSCs, which collectively accounted for about 95 percent of individuals in critical medical career fields.[14] These included 14 officer AFSCs and six enlisted AFSCs.[15] For each AFSC and policy combination, we simulated monthly results spanning a 20-year period. For purposes of reporting results, we grouped locations into five categories: CONUS Tier 1 locations, CONUS Tier 2 locations, other OCONUS locations, Alaska and Hawaii locations, and WestPac locations (see Appendix A).

We begin by reporting the impact of the policies on manning, tour length, and assignment sequences and on average proficiency for two sample officer and enlisted AFSCs: Aerospace Medical Service, 4N0X1, and Critical Care Clinical Nurse, 46NXE. We also report how the policies affect proficiency for all critical medical AFSCs. In the tables and figures that follow, "Duration" refers to reduced tour lengths at low-volume locations, "Priority" refers to assignment sequencing, and "Manning" refers to the use of military personnel at high-volume locations and nonmilitary personnel at low-volume locations.

Impact of Assignment Policies on Manning, Tour Length, and Assignment Sequences

Although the first-order effects related to proficiency of these new assignment policies are fixed, they may produce unexpected second-order effects. To examine these effects, we used the simulation results to determine the impact of assignment policies on manning, tour lengths, and assignment sequences. Additionally, it was unclear whether policies involving assignment sequences were even possible given current authorizations by AFSC and location. Finally, the effects of these policies on proficiency are mediated through their impact on manning, tour lengths, and assignment sequences, and so it was important to first establish these proximal outcomes.

In the baseline scenario, 48 percent of 4N0X1 assignments and 78 percent of 46NXE assignments are at CONUS Tier 1 locations (comprising 2,541 and 294 individuals, respectively). For policies that increased military personnel at Tier 1 locations (i.e., columns in Table 4.1 that contain "Manning" in the title), these values increased to 57 percent and 90 percent (comprising 2,978 and 336 individuals, respectively).[16] The increases were offset by a proportional decrease in manning at CONUS Tier 2 locations. The average tour length is three years at some WestPac

---

[14] AFSCs were drawn from the list of critical career fields presented in Chapter 2 and were further disaggregated to the shredout level.

[15] Officer AFSCs were 42GX, 44EXA, 44MX, 45AX, 45BX, 45SX, 46NX, 46NXE, 46NXG, 46NXJ, 46SX, 46YXH, 46YXM, and 48RX; enlisted AFSCs were 4H0X1, 4N0X1, 4N0X1C, 4N0X1F, 4N1X1, and 4N1X1C.

[16] We increased manning at Tier 1 locations by 25 percent (up to a maximum of 110 percent of authorizations). One could raise the ceiling further to increase the overall percentage of individuals at Tier 1 locations.

locations (Andersen Air Force Base, Kadena Air Base, Misawa Air Base, and Yokota Air Base), and one year at others (Kunsan Air Base and Osan Air Base). These differences reflect policies that set accompanied and unaccompanied tour lengths by location.

For policies that limited WestPac assignment durations (i.e., columns in Table 4.1 that contain "Duration"), tour length was fixed to 12 months at all WestPac locations and tour length at all other locations was unaffected. Table 4.1 shows the percentage of assignments to each category that came from Tier 1 locations. In the baseline scenario, 51 percent of 4N0X1 assignments and 77 percent of 46NXE assignments to WestPac were from Tier 1 locations. For policy options that prioritized assignments (i.e., columns in Table 4.1 that contain "priority" in the title), these values increased to 84 percent or more. The values did not reach 100 percent because not enough individuals were available from Tier 1 locations during some months in the simulation. The increased flow of individuals from Tier 1 locations to WestPac was offset by reduced flow of individuals from Tier 1 locations to all other categories.

Table 4.1. Percentage of Assignments Originating from Tier 1 Locations

AFSC	Category	Baseline	Duration	Priority	Manning	Duration and Priority	Duration and Manning	Priority and Manning	Duration, Priority, and Manning
4N0X1	CONUS Tier 1	60%	58%	59%	62%	52%	61%	60%	57%
	CONUS Tier 2	70%	59%	62%	83%	52%	62%	75%	55%
	OCONUS	52%	49%	48%	59%	38%	58%	54%	45%
	Alaska and Hawaii	58%	54%	53%	75%	38%	61%	63%	45%
	WestPac	51%	49%	100%	60%	84%	54%	100%	84%
46NXE	CONUS Tier 1	66%	65%	65%	80%	62%	78%	78%	74%
	CONUS Tier 2	80%	79%	82%	97%	78%	92%	91%	88%
	OCONUS	85%	80%	79%	95%	71%	86%	92%	89%
	Alaska and Hawaii	—	—	—	—	—	—	—	—
	WestPac	77%	71%	96%	82%	94%	84%	96%	96%

NOTE: Values are not shown for 46NXE assignments to Alaska and Hawaii because there were too few positions at those locations to generate reliable estimates.

Aside from the direct effects of assignment sequencing shown in Table 4.1, the other policy options indirectly affected assignment flows:

- When WestPac assignment durations were reduced, fewer assignments to non-WestPac locations came from Tier 1 locations. This is because reducing WestPac assignment durations increased WestPac turnover, which non-WestPac locations absorbed.
- When Tier 1 manning was increased, more assignments to all locations came from Tier 1 locations. This is because more individuals at Tier 1 locations were available for assignment.

Proficiency Results for Two Sample Air Force Specialty Codes

In this simulation model, an individual's proficiency depends on their location, their proficiency when they arrived at the location, and the number of months that they spent at the location. Figure 4.3 shows average proficiency by location and policy combination. Proficiency was greatest at CONUS Tier 1 locations—that is, locations where individuals build proficiency. In the baseline scenario (red bars), proficiency was comparable across the remaining location categories.

Figure 4.3. Average Proficiency by Location Category

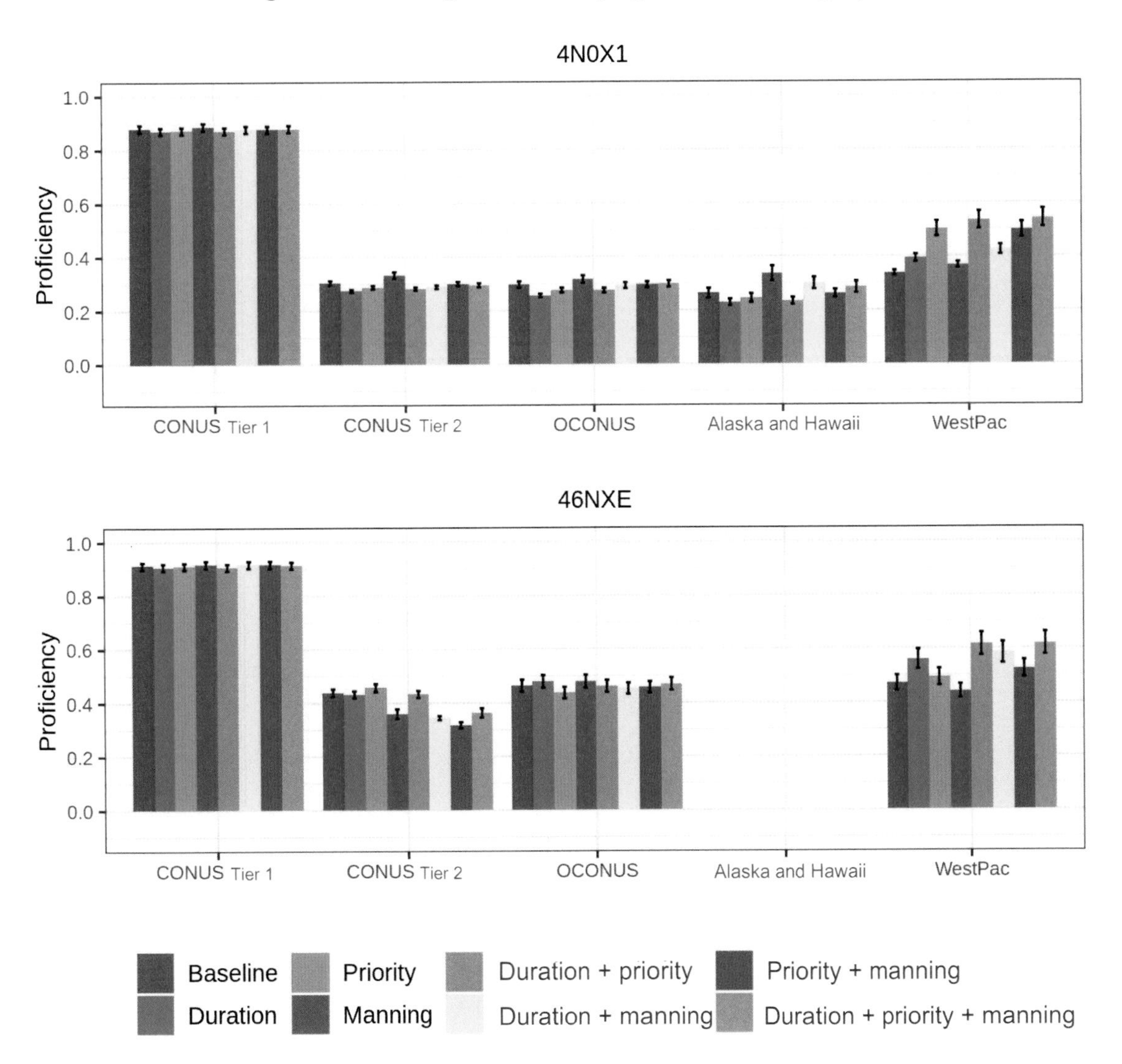

NOTE: Values are not shown for 46NXE assignments in Alaska and Hawaii because there were too few 46NXE positions at those locations to reliably estimate proficiency.

The effects of the policy options were most apparent for WestPac, which is expected given that the policies were tailored for this location, and varied by AFSC. Reducing assignment duration or prioritizing assignments of individuals from Tier 1 locations to WestPac increased proficiency relative to the baseline scenario (blue and green bars, respectively) for both AFSCs. However, the benefits of sequencing were greatest for 4N0X1 assignments, whereas the benefits of reducing assignment duration were greatest for 46NXE assignments. This is because in the baseline, a relatively low percentage of 4N0X1 assignments to WestPac were from Tier 1 locations; thus, prioritizing flows had a large benefit. In contrast, a relatively high percentage of 46NXE assignments to WestPac were from Tier 1 locations; thus, reducing the duration of time for skill decay to occur had a large benefit.

For both AFSCs, prioritizing assignment sequences or reducing assignment durations caused a slight decrease in proficiency at non-WestPac locations.[17] Increasing manning at Tier 1 locations also increased proficiency for 4N0X1 assignments relative to the baseline scenario; the benefits extended to all locations. Combining policy options tended to produce larger benefits than did using policies in isolation. Finally, increasing Tier 1 manning offset the negative effects of other policy options on non-WestPac locations.

There are costs associated with implementing these policies. Decreasing tour lengths at WestPac locations is estimated to increase the number of permanent change-of-station moves by approximately 30 percent, resulting in the need for additional PCS funding.. Increasing Tier 1 manning requires additional civilian or contractor personnel at Tier 2 locations. For the simulated example AFSC assignments, 437 civilian or contractor Aerospace Medical Service personnel and 42 critical care clinical nurses would need to be employed. Assignment sequencing, if feasible, is the least costly policy option from a workforce perspective.

Proficiency Results Across All Simulated Critical Medical Air Force Specialty Codes

In our final analysis, we examined the effects of assignment policies individually and in combination on average proficiency for all critical medical AFSCs. Figure 4.4 shows proficiency at WestPac locations for the 20 largest AFSCs. Each tile represents simulation results for an AFSC and policy or combination of policies, with the tile colors indicating the average proficiency, ranging from lowest to highest. Tiles with dark borders denote the largest increase in proficiency for a policy relative to the baseline in cases with one additional assignment policy (the second through fourth columns) and with two additional assignment policies (the fifth through seventh columns).

When we considered each policy in isolation, reducing assignment duration was most effective for improving proficiency relative to the baseline scenario for 12 AFSCs, and prioritizing Tier 1 assignments was most effective for the remaining eight AFSCs. The effectiveness of the policies depended on AFSC-specific assignment dynamics. For example, in the baseline case, 51 percent of 4N0X1 assignments to WestPac were from Tier 1 locations, whereas nearly all 44MX assignments were from Tier 1 locations. As a result, prioritizing assignments was very beneficial for 4N0X1 assignments (i.e., a 16-percent improvement relative to the baseline), whereas it had little effect for 44MX assignments (i.e., a 2-percent improvement). However, because most 44MX assignments had high proficiency when they arrived at WestPac locations, substantial skill decay occurred during those assignments. As a result, reducing assignment duration was very beneficial for 44MX assignments (i.e., a 12-percent improvement relative to baseline), whereas it was less beneficial for 4N0X1 assignments (i.e., a 6-percent improvement).

---

[17] The decrease arose from the reduced flow of individuals from Tier 1 locations to non-WestPac locations.

Figure 4.4. Average Proficiency of Individuals in the Western Pacific, by Air Force Specialty Code and Simulation

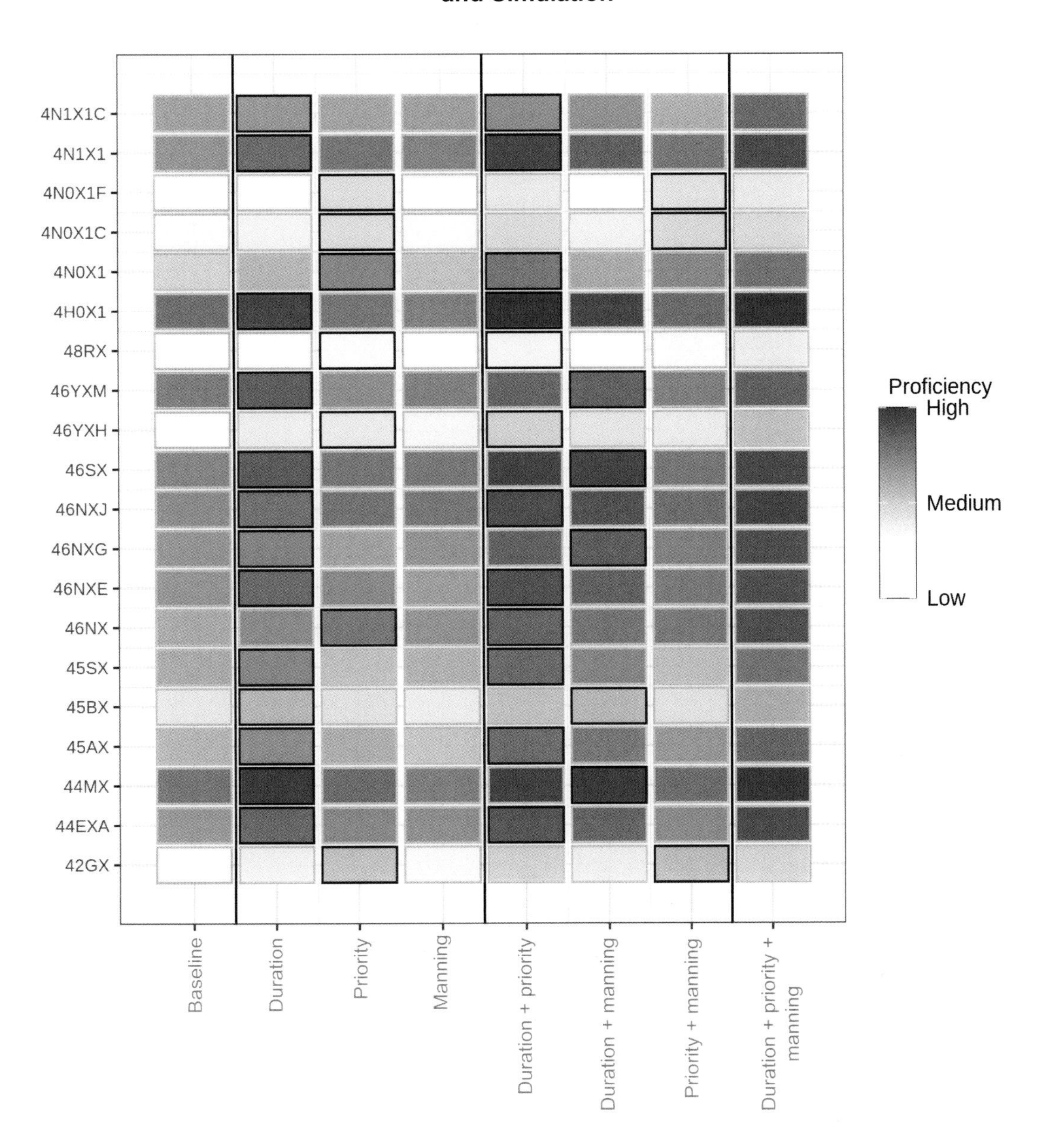

When we considered pairs of assignment policy options, reducing assignment duration while prioritizing assignments was most effective for 13 AFSCs, reducing assignment duration while increasing Tier 1 manning was most effective for four AFSCs, and prioritizing assignments while increasing Tier 1 manning was most effective for the remaining three AFSCs. Once again, the effectiveness of the combinations depended on AFSC-specific assignment dynamics. For example, prioritizing assignments increased the proficiency of individuals in the 4N0X1 career field when they were assigned to WestPac. This option increased the potential for skill decay to occur during assignments. As a result, reducing 4N0X1 assignment durations *after* prioritizing sequences was more beneficial than simply reducing assignment durations.

Combining all three assignment policy options produced a meaningful benefit for certain AFSCs such as 46NX assignments (i.e., a 20-percent improvement relative to baseline). Given the number of 46NX assignments at Tier 1 locations, it was not always possible to meet the demand to assign individuals from Tier 1 locations to WestPac. By increasing manning at Tier 1 locations, it became possible to assign more individuals from Tier 1 locations to WestPac even while reducing WestPac tour lengths.

All of these results held for a wide range of parameter values for the rate of skill acquisition and skill decay, with the caveat that the benefits of shortened assignments were even greater for higher values of skill decay (see Appendix A).

Chapter Summary

The results described in this chapter reveal four primary findings:

1. Reducing WestPac assignment durations or prioritizing the flow of individuals from Tier 1 locations to WestPac reduced the flow of individuals from Tier 1 locations to non-WestPac locations. This had a negative effect on clinical proficiency at those locations. In effect, it is a zero-sum game. However, the size of the effect was very small because WestPac constitutes only a small percentage of total AFMS manning.
2. Reducing assignment duration is most beneficial when individuals are proficient when they arrive at WestPac. This is already the case for some AFSCs where all or most assignments to WestPac are from Tier 1 locations, and this can be accomplished for other AFSCs by prioritizing the flow of individuals from Tier 1 locations to WestPac.
3. The increased demand for assignments created by reducing WestPac tour length may exceed the number of individuals available from Tier 1 locations. Increasing manning at Tier 1 locations may help to meet this demand.
4. Increasing manning at Tier 1 locations may also offset the negative effects of other policy options at non-WestPac locations.

Given that the effects of the assignment policies varied somewhat by AFSC, the AFMS should tailor the selection of assignment policies by AFSC if it chooses to pursue them. The implementation of these assignment policies may require changes to DoD and Department of the Air Force (DAF) policy and will need to be synchronized with existing assignment policies.

The benefits of the assignment policies may appear modest. In a sense, this is because the options are defensive: they seek to create a buffer to ensure a minimal level of currency given some amount of skill decay or they seek to reduce the potential for skill decay to occur. Alternative activities, such as training that reverses skill decay, would be even more effective at maximizing readiness at WestPac locations.

Chapter 5. A Framework for Matching Personnel to Readiness Activities

Ensuring that the medical force is ready to go to war is the responsibility of the Air Force as a whole. Consequently, it is in the interest of the Air Force Surgeon General to have a holistic view of the readiness of all personnel across AFSCs and of the different readiness building activities that each might undertake. This in turn would enable the Air Force Surgeon General to identify which AFSCs require more attention and which activities require increased investment.

In this chapter we present a possible approach by which a headquarters-type entity, such as the Air Force Surgeon General's staff or the Air Force Medical Readiness Agency, might catalog the needs of different types of personnel, catalog the characteristics of different types of readiness building activities and policies, and match one to the other. Using PACAF as an example, our purpose is to show the type of analysis an AFMS entity could carry out and, in particular, how assignment policies such as those discussed in Chapter 4 could be considered as part of a holistic set of readiness building strategies.

Our prototype framework for assigning personnel to readiness activities contains three components.[1] In the first component, personnel are scored based on select characteristics and assigned a priority score. In the second component, readiness building activities are rated on the degree to which they enhance readiness for trauma and critical care. The third component provides a systematic approach to matching personnel to activities. The goal is to achieve the highest level of readiness possible across the AFMS.

Scoring Personnel

We begin by assigning a priority score to different types of personnel based on the characteristics shown in the first five columns in Table 5.1. The primary distinction we make among personnel is between WestPac, CONUS, and Alaska and Hawaii. These personnel types are then subdivided into surgical AFSCs, critical care AFSCs, nonsurgical and noncritical care AFSCs, and IDMTs.

---

[1] These three components were derived from the relationships illustrated in the logic model described in Appendix C. The logic model we constructed depicts how people, facilities, and programs combine to produce medical personnel who are ready for their wartime missions.

Table 5.1. The Scheme for Prioritizing Personnel

Type of Personnel	Proximity to Fight	Sensitivity to Skill Loss	Likelihood of No Backup	Sensitivity to Teamwork	Priority Score (sum of *Yes* answers)	Ease of Embedding
WestPac						
Surgical	Yes	Yes		Yes	3	Hard, or not possible
Critical care	Yes	Yes			2	Hard, or not possible
Nonsurgical and noncritical care	Yes				1	Hard, or not possible
IDMT	Yes	Yes	Yes		3	Hard, or not possible
CONUS						
Surgical		Yes		Yes	2	Easy
Critical care		Yes			1	Easy
Nonsurgical and noncritical care					0	Moderate
IDMT		Yes	Yes		2	Hard
Alaska and Hawaii						
Surgical		Yes		Yes	2	Easy
Critical care		Yes			1	Easy
Nonsurgical and noncritical care					0	Moderate
IDMT		Yes	Yes		2	Hard

The criteria used in this prioritization scheme are as follows:

- *Proximity to fight.* Those who need to be ready to "fight tonight" should be kept at a higher degree of readiness than those who do not. This means, for example, that WestPac personnel would be of a higher priority than CONUS personnel. Or priorities might be assigned to other categories of personnel. For example, special operations teams, those postured to be the initial follow-on forces for U.S. Indo-Pacific Command, or those deploying to other combat areas might be considered of higher priority. "Yes" indicates personnel types who are proximal to the fight.
- *Sensitivity to skill loss.* Some AFSCs may be considered more skill based, while other AFSCs are more knowledge based. Conversations with medical personnel suggest that surgery and critical care AFSCs are more skill based and thus sensitive to skill loss. IDMTs may also fall into this category. "Yes" indicates that the type of personnel is sensitive to skill loss.
- *Likelihood of no backup.* Some AFSCs may be required to operate without backup. IDMTs and some forward surgical teams, for example, may have to function alone in austere environments without support from other medical personnel or rapid aeromedical evacuation. "Yes" indicates personnel types who are likely to have no backup.

- *Sensitivity to teamwork.* Teamwork is always important, but some functions may be more sensitive to good teamwork than others. Surgical teams and Critical Care Air Transport Teams could fall into this category. "Yes" indicates personnel types for which teamwork plays an important role.[2]

The final two columns are used in the framework to match personnel to readiness building activities:

- *Priority score.* The priority score is calculated by summing up the number of "Yes" entries in each row. In the table, for example, WestPac surgical AFSCs total three yeses, while CONUS AFSCs not involved in surgery or critical care total zero. A higher score indicates higher priority for readiness building activities.
- *Ease of embedding.* This column is used to note which types of personnel are harder to place in civilian trauma centers, a factor that will be considered in our eventual matching algorithm. We rated surgical AFSCs as being easy to place in civilian hospitals. IDMTs are rated as hard to place based on the incompatibility between IDMT training levels and civilian certification equivalency. Personnel assigned to WestPac would not be able to participate in activities that involve embedding in CONUS trauma centers.

Rating Readiness Building Activities

Next we score the readiness building activities using the scheme depicted in Table 5.2. The rating here is not intended as a way of prioritizing the activities, as if one would be better than another for all situations. Rather, the focus is on cataloging key characteristics of each activity to facilitate matching appropriate activities to different types of personnel. The rows of Table 5.2 are the training and practice activities listed in Table 3.1. Because the assignment policies described in Chapter 4 are of a different nature, we do not include them in the table, but they are considered within the overall framework.

Table 5.2. The Scheme for Rating Readiness Building Activities

Activity	Fraction of Time Spent Practicing on Trauma	Fraction of Time Spent on Critical Care	Fraction of Time Spent Away from MTF	Feasible for WestPac Personnel?	Relative Ease of Expansion Given Manpower, Resource, and Coordination Constraints
Attending C-STARS before or during PACAF assignment	Some	Some	Some	Yes	Easier
Attending a trauma training course	Some	Little	Little	Yes	Easier

[2] The criteria were selected based on information gathered during stakeholder discussion, from trauma subject-matter experts, and from our literature review. The project sponsor agreed that these were important considerations. Additional criteria may be added after further analysis.

Activity	Fraction of Time Spent Practicing on Trauma	Fraction of Time Spent on Critical Care	Fraction of Time Spent Away from MTF	Feasible for WestPac Personnel?	Relative Ease of Expansion Given Manpower, Resource, and Coordination Constraints
Attending advanced simulation training	Some	Little	Little	Yes	Moderate
Practicing in a trauma center MTF	High	High	None	No	Harder
Practicing intermittently at a higher-volume MTF via a TDY within-skill exchange program	Some	Some	None	Yes	Easier
Embedding at a civilian Level 1 trauma center	Highest	Highest	All	No	Harder
Embedding at a civilian Level 1 trauma center as a C-STARS cadre	High	High	All	No	Harder
Practicing intermittently at a civilian Level 1 trauma center	Some	Some	Some	No	Moderate
Embedding at a VAMC	None	Moderate	All	No	Harder
Embedding at a VAMC as a cadre	None	Moderate	All	No	Harder
Practicing intermittently at a VAMC	None	Some	Some	No	Moderate
Using ODE to practice intermittently at a civilian trauma center or intensive care unit	Some	Some	None	No	Easier

The characteristics used to rate each activity are as follows:

- *Fraction of time spent practicing on trauma cases.* Activities differ in the amount of time individuals spend honing their trauma skills. Full-time activities such as embedding at a civilian Level 1 trauma center or assignment to an MTF that is a trauma center would provide high trauma training. In contrast, embedding at a VA would provide no trauma training. Part-time readiness building activities such as intermittent duty or ODE offer some practice; others that involve simulation rather than the care of actual patients would offer a little practice in trauma care.
- *Fraction of time spent practicing on critical care cases.* This criterion is similar to time spent on trauma cases but focuses on critical care. The difference is that activities involving VA score higher here than they did on trauma.
- *Fraction of time spent away from an MTF.* The downside of spending large amounts of time in training or at a civilian hospital is that it takes the medical personnel away from their duties providing care to service members and other beneficiaries at the MTF. Thus, the time away from an MTF is one cost of an activity.
- *Feasibility for WestPac personnel.* WestPac personnel can participate in some activities if travel funding is available, and they can be sufficiently backfilled. Other activities,

especially the embed options, are effectively impossible (absent the development of partnerships in Japan or South Korea).

- *Relative ease of expansion.* The activities on our list were designed based on existing programs to ensure feasibility. However, existing programs may require expansion to accommodate larger numbers of participants. We judged expanding the number of students in training courses and simulations to be relatively easy compared with other options, recognizing there would be cost involved. Expanding the number of people embedded full-time in partner hospitals (civilian Level 1 trauma or VA) was deemed to be more difficult due to the need to develop additional partnership locations. Developing an MTF into a trauma center would be even harder still, due to the need to build up the staff and capability of the MTF to meet the necessary standards and the need for buy-in from the local community's trauma system.

Matching Personnel to Readiness Activities

Having prioritized the different types of personnel and rated the different types of readiness activities, we developed an algorithm for matching types of personnel to activities, which is illustrated in Figure 5.1. Starting with the personnel scored with the highest priority (from the priority scores assigned from Table 5.1), we proceed through a series of questions.

Figure 5.1. Algorithm for Matching Types of Personnel to Readiness Activities

Start: next type of personnel on priority list

WestPac or other remote location?
Yes:
- Prioritize for C-STARS/SMART rotation before and/or during PACAF assignment
- Supplement with additional training (simulations, traveling training teams, etc.)
- Practice at higher-volume MTF via a TDY within-skill exchange program
- Use short duration assignments and prioritize gaining personnel from Tier 1 locations

No → AFSC hard to embed in civilian hospitals?
Yes:
- When assigned to MTF, supplement with additional training (simulations, exercises, etc.)
- Prioritize for C-STARS/SMART rotation (i.e., second-highest priority)
- Encourage ODE to gain additional trauma experience

No → Billets available at Level 1 trauma centers?
Yes:
- Embed in Level 1 trauma center, with or without cadre duties

No → Does MTF have patients of sufficient acuity?
Yes:
- When assigned to MTF, supplement with additional training (simulations, exercises, etc.)

No → Full-time nontrauma more useful than part-time trauma?
Yes → Billets available at VAMC?
Yes:
- Embed in VAMC, with or without cadre duties

No → Partnerships available at local hospitals?
Yes:
- When assigned to MTF, supplement with additional training (simulations, exercises, etc.)
- TAA to do intermittent duty at Level 1 local trauma center, or else at VAMC

No:
- Assign to MTF, supplement with additional training (simulations, exercises, etc.)
- Prioritize for C-STARS/SMART rotation (i.e., third-highest priority)
- Encourage ODE to gain additional trauma experience

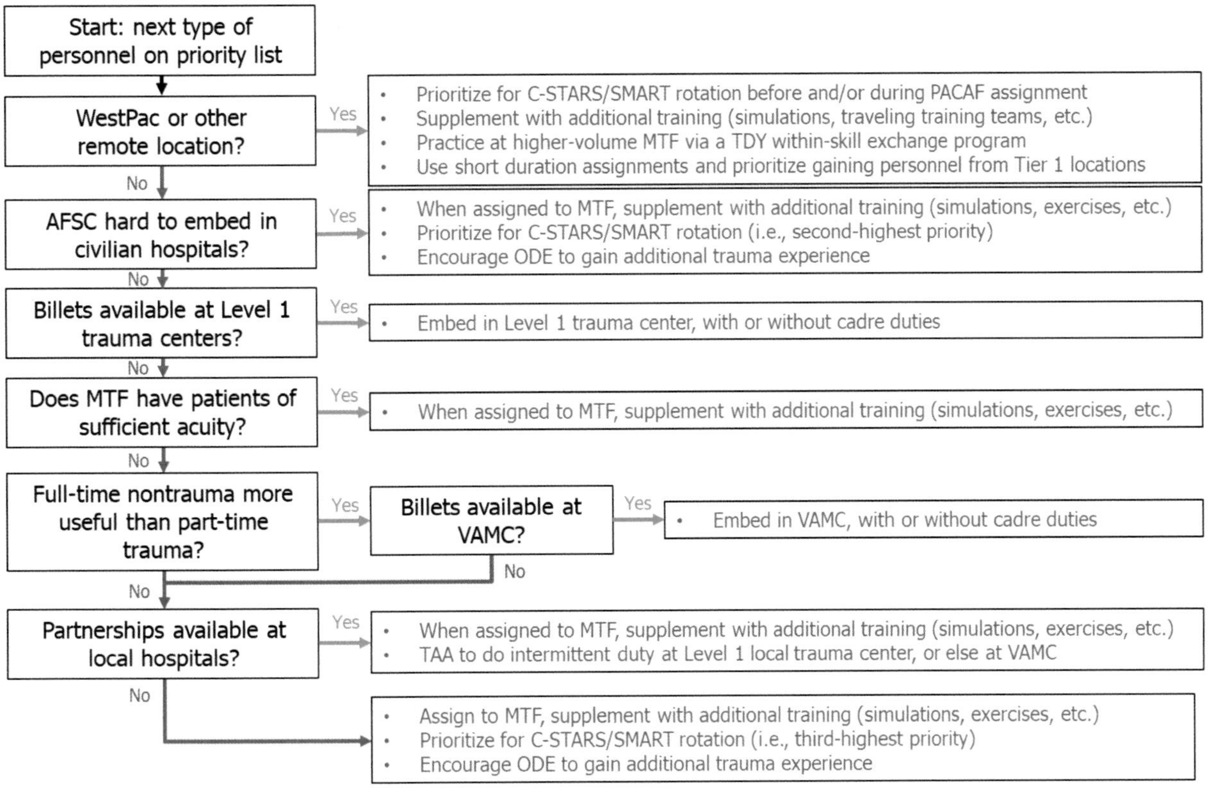

Are these personnel in WestPac or another remote location? This first step in the algorithm will be the one of most interest to PACAF, but it also illustrates the importance of taking an enterprise-wide view of readiness activities. If the personnel being considered are to be based in WestPac or some other forward or remote location, then these personnel will not be able to take part in any embedding activities or work intermittently in civilian hospitals. Therefore, they should receive priority for *attending C-STARS before or during PACAF*. At their WestPac assignment, they could supplement their work with additional training, such as participation in a *trauma course* or *simulation training* or practice in a *TDY within-skill exchange program*. In addition, the various assignment policies described in Chapter 4 could be used to bolster readiness of WestPac personnel.

We note that many of these readiness activities and policies are out of the control of PACAF. For example, PACAF may prioritize sending WestPac personnel to C-STARS, but USAFSAM would also need to prioritize WestPac personnel for receiving spots in the rotations. Similarly, the various assignment policies are not under control of PACAF or even the Air Force Surgeon General but require coordination across Air Force agencies. Thus, an enterprise-wide view is required to help PACAF meet its requirement for ready medical personnel.

Is the AFSC hard to embed in civilian hospitals? If yes, such personnel would be assigned to an MTF and attend training courses and simulations. They should receive the second-highest priority for attendance at C-STARS. They could also pursue ODE to supplement their MTF work, though we note that AFSCs that are difficult to embed at a hospital may find it similarly difficult to find ODE at a hospital.

Are positions available at Level 1 trauma centers? Personnel who are not assigned to WestPac and not difficult to embed in civilian trauma centers would be *embedded at a civilian Level 1 trauma center* if positions are available. The number of positions available is a function of the number of partnerships that exist and a decision by the Air Force on how many personnel to allow to work outside MTFs. If positions are not available, this shortage would be a signal to identify more embed positions and to develop more partnership locations.

Does the MTF have patients of sufficient acuity? If full-time embedded positions in Level 1 trauma centers are no longer available, then personnel would be assigned to high-acuity MTFs and supplement their practice with training courses and simulation. *Expanding trauma care at MTFs* would help ensure that personnel at MTFs have the high-acuity patients needed to keep their skills sharp.

Would full-time, high-acuity nontrauma assignments be preferable to part-time trauma assignments? If the positions in high-volume, high-acuity MTFs are filled, whether personnel would be assigned to work full-time with high-acuity nontrauma patients or work part-time with trauma patients would be determined based on the AFSC. If working full-time with high-acuity nontrauma patients is an acceptable trade-off, then personnel can *embed at VAMCs*, assuming positions are available.

Are partnerships available at local hospitals? If working a part-time trauma assignment is preferred over working a full-time, high-acuity nontrauma assignment, or if positions are not available at VA hospitals, then personnel would be assigned to MTFs. If partnerships are available at local hospitals, then the MTF work could be supplemented by *practicing intermittently at civilian Level 1 trauma centers*. If there are no opportunities at trauma centers, then the personnel could *practice intermittently at VAMCs*. If partnerships are unavailable, personnel can augment their MTF practice with *traveling trauma courses* and *simulation training*. These personnel would be prioritized for C-STARS or SMART, though with lower priority than those assigned to WestPac or those who are difficult to embed.

After matching the highest-priority personnel, the process repeats with the next group of personnel on the priority list until all types of personnel are placed.

Chapter Summary

The prototype framework we describe in this chapter assigns priorities to different types of personnel and matches them with activities according to their priority ranking, constraints on personnel, and constraints on activities. It also demonstrates the interconnectedness between readiness requirements unique to particular AFSCs, theaters, or missions, such as those specific to WestPac; and the collection of training activities, practice activities, and assignment policies that are available, including those that are not under the control of PACAF.

We recognize that others may disagree with how we scored personnel or rated the activities and could change the scoring and come up with a different outcome. That said, using this type of framework would enable the AFMS to take a holistic view of different strategies for building readiness and systematically employ them for different types of personnel.

Chapter 6. Findings and Recommendations

PACAF's ability to provide trauma and critical care is dependent on the proficiency and readiness of the personnel currently assigned in critical medical specialties in PACAF, those who will be assigned to PACAF in the future, and those who might deploy in times of conflict. Therefore, activities that build currency and readiness across the AFMS are beneficial to PACAF, which is reflected in our research and recommendations.

Moreover, medical personnel assigned to MTFs care for a relatively young and healthy patient population and have minimal exposure to trauma and critical care cases during their day-to-day practice. As a result, the knowledge and skills that medical personnel practicing at MTFs will need to save lives during emergency situations are likely to decay. To improve the medical readiness of personnel who will be called on to "fight tonight," a broader portfolio of readiness building activities and a systematic approach to assigning personnel is necessary. Preceding the decision to resource these activities, it may be necessary to decide whether the priority is deployable medical teams that are proficient in delivering trauma and critical care in an austere environment or instead in-garrison health care.

Findings

We identified a number of issues affecting the readiness of critical medical personnel in WestPac and the broader AFMS:

- Given the strategic importance of the region, relatively few personnel in critical medical specialties are assigned to WestPac locations, and some specialties are undermanned. Even though these personnel tend to be more experienced, on average, than those in CONUS locations, undermanning combined with skill decay in such a remote region can have a significant impact on readiness—particularly in responding to the need to "fight tonight."
- Deployments have been opportunities to develop proficiency for AFSCs, but these opportunities are declining. The majority of critical AFSCs were deployed for less than 5 percent of their total time served during the three-year period from 2018 through 2020. The impact on proficiency needs to be better understood, and other options to develop proficiency and readiness need to be utilized.
- The AFMS uses CMRP checklists to identify readiness requirements for medical professionals and evaluate the readiness of these professionals to provide care. But these checklists do not fully function as intended, in part because the requirements are not well defined for all AFSCs. Many lack wartime requirements, others prescribe requirements that fall short of civilian standards, and options for meeting requirements are assumed to be generally equivalent when in fact they vary considerably in experiences gained. As a result, there is no effective standard against which to measure readiness, measure improvements in knowledge or skills, or identify areas of concern.

- We could identify no single office or organization with visibility over the types of readiness activities currently being used throughout MAJCOMS and the MTFs, lessons learned, or investments being made and required. As a result, it appears that sharing information on effective readiness initiatives occurs primarily on an ad hoc basis.

A range of options exist to help improve critical medical personnel's readiness via developing a portfolio of readiness building activities:

- Training activities are perhaps the easiest options to increase proficiency because they can be focused directly on trauma and critical care, have low manpower costs and time commitment, and require little coordination outside the Air Force. Some options, such as increasing advanced simulation training, would require additional investment to expand opportunities for participation.
- Readiness activities in the practice category include a wide variety of options for placing medical personnel in settings that require more-intensive patient care than the typical MTF. These activities vary in cost, time commitment required, ease of implementation (depending on location of personnel), and other factors. The different characteristics of these options accommodate the requirements of different AFSCs and specialties. The activities identified during our research offer a robust set of options that can be evaluated for use across the AFMS.
- Our investigations showed that some assignment policies could contribute to readiness for WestPac without having a negative effect on other locations. Shortening tours and tailoring assignment sequencing can mitigate skill decay and promote higher levels of readiness across the critical medical specialties. Combining these options, along with using nonmilitary personnel at low-volume locations, produced a meaningful increase in proficiency for several AFSCs.
- Readiness building activities may be most beneficial when matched to different types of personnel according to their priority ranking, constraints on participation, and constraints on activities. Using a systematic framework would enable the AFMS to take a holistic view of different strategies for building readiness and assign them to different types of personnel.

Recommendations

The Air Force should treat the readiness of medical personnel as an enterprise problem requiring an enterprise solution. This effort should include considering the role of DHA with respect to military treatment facilities (MTFs) in setting policy, determining force and capability distribution, and in directing funding. Currently, readiness tends to be addressed at the local level. While many good ideas and approaches are being employed, these are not shared in a way that they can be more widely applied. Moreover, readiness issues cut across units, career fields, and MAJCOMS and require actions that go beyond those that any one entity can undertake. To implement this recommendation, the AFMS needs to undertake the following:

- **Ensure an organizational entity has the authority, resources, and obligation to maintain an enterprise-wide view of the proficiency and readiness of medical**

personnel. This entity would monitor the readiness of personnel across units, MTFs, and career fields in cooperation with the respective clinical consultants; monitor the state of readiness programs underway; and offer assistance to MTFs and MAJCOMS in implementing and facilitating readiness building activities, such as establishing agreements with civilian and VA hospitals.

- **Develop consistent metrics for reviewing readiness levels across critical medical AFSCs that can be used to monitor personnel in different types of assignments.** As a first step, increase the specificity and consistency of CMRP checklists, which set forth basic readiness requirements for all AFSCs. Improving these checklists could improve desired outcomes—that is, current and ready medical personnel. As a second step, update the readiness requirements in CMRP checklists with readiness activities provided as options for each AFSC, and with improved metrics for monitoring readiness, such as a mature KSA metric. Particular attention should be paid to those assigned forward or postured to deploy forward to potential combat areas such as WestPac.
- **Take a portfolio approach to employing and developing readiness building activities.** The AFMS needs to build a catalog of readiness building activities and track the unique requirements of each AFSC and specialty. In doing so, the AFMS can determine gaps in capabilities, thus identifying which types of personnel require more training and practice and where additional investments in readiness building activities should be made. Activities that confer the greatest readiness—for example, embedding at a civilian Level 1 trauma center or expanding trauma care at an MTF—are likely to be a scarce resource, with low availability or high cost. If this resource is allocated through uncoordinated local decisionmaking that fails to account for the enterprise-wide readiness needs of the AFMS and forward locations like WestPac, there is a risk that those personnel and AFSCs with the greatest need for high-quality readiness activities will not receive them. By taking a portfolio approach, the AFMS can better match the right activities to the right population based on the requirements of each AFSC.

The AFMS, in collaboration with the AFPC, should view assignments over the course of a career as a key component in the development of the proficiency and readiness of its personnel. Taking an enterprise-wide view, assignment policies can contribute to building and maintaining readiness over time. Potential policies include reducing tour lengths at low-volume locations, including WestPac; potentially limiting extensions at Tier 1 locations; sequencing assignments to maintain or improve proficiency; and using military personnel at high-volume locations and nonmilitary personnel at low-volume locations. Implementation may involve increased manpower and operational costs and require changes to DAF and DoD policy. In addition, new policies will need to be synchronized with existing assignment policies, such as voluntary tour extensions at overseas locations.

PACAF should continue to advocate for activities and policies that enhance proficiency of wartime skills and readiness for potential conflict. Because of the criticality of the Indo-Pacific Command region, PACAF's requirements for ready medical personnel should be a priority. However, many readiness building activities are not available to WestPac personnel due to their location. This constraint, and a reliance on follow-on forces for WestPac, necessitate an AFMS-wide focus on readiness for the potential conflict. PACAF must continue to make its readiness requirements clear and compelling. PACAF's efforts to identify capability gaps for ensuring operational readiness must be visible to the Air Force Surgeon General.

The AFMS should undertake a comprehensive assessment of the requirements for medical simulation across the spectrum of modes, levels of complexity, and needed outcomes, to include infrastructure and support. Of all the readiness building activities available to personnel assigned to WestPac locations, simulation is the least well defined and offers opportunities for remote locations. It is unclear whether ongoing Air Force efforts to acquire medical simulation systems will be available for personnel in WestPac or whether the purposes of these systems are best suited for the specialties and skills required to maintain readiness in the PACAF theater. Further, to be most effective, fielding of these simulation systems must include planned and funded maintenance and upgrades, personnel experienced in their use, and leadership to ensure simulations provide effective training.

Appendix A. Assignment Policy Modeling and Simulation Details

In this appendix we provide additional details on the analytic methods used in our analysis of the personnel assignments discussed in Chapter 4. This includes details about the statistical model of the assignment system, the computational cognitive model of skill acquisition and retention, and the interplay between cognitive model parameters and proficiency results.

Location Classifications

Table A.1 contains regional and tier classifications by location.

Table A.1. Regional and Proficiency Tier Classifications by Base and Location

Region	Tier	Bases and Locations
CONUS	Tier 1	Baltimore, Beaufort, Bethesda, Birmingham, Bremerton, Brooks City, Camp Pendleton, Cincinnati, Eglin Air Force Base, El Paso, Fort Belvoir, Fort Benning, Fort Bragg, Fort Campbell, Fort Carson, Fort Gordon, Fort Hood, Fort Leonard Wood, Fort Sam Houston, Jacksonville, Joint Base Langley-Eustis, Joint Base San Antonio–Camp Bullis, Joint Base San Antonio–Lackland, Keesler Air Force Base, Madigan Army Medical Center, Naval Base San Diego, Nellis Air Force Base, Portsmouth Naval Shipyard, St. Louis, Travis Air Force Base, Walter Reed Army Medical Center, Wright-Patterson Air Force Base
	Tier 2	All other CONUS bases and locations
OCONUS	Tier 2	All OCONUS locations not included in Alaska and Hawaii or WestPac
Alaska and Hawaii	Tier 1	Tripler General
Alaska and Hawaii	Tier 2	Eielson, Elmhurst, Elmendorf-Richardson, Pearl Harbor–Hickam, and all other locations in Alaska and Hawaii
WestPac	Tier 1	Okinawa
	Tier 2	Andersen, Daegu, Diego Garcia, Kadena, Kunsan, Misawa, Osan, Yokota, and all other locations in WestPac

Inputs to the Statistical Model of Assignments

The statistical model of the assignment system took four sets of probabilities for each AFSC: (1) initial assignment location for new accessions, (2) assignment sequence, (3) monthly assignment probability, and (4) monthly separation probability. We calculated these inputs using officer and enlisted personnel files that covered CY 2010–CY 2020. We use the enlisted career field Aerospace Medical Service, 4N0X1, to illustrate these inputs.

To calculate initial assignment location for new accessions, we identified when everyone first entered the force. We then computed the percentage of initial assignments by location. For 4N0X1 assignments, more than 95 percent occurred at three locations: Fort Sam Houston (75 percent), Sheppard Air Force Base (11 percent), and Joint Base San Antonio–Lackland (10 percent).

To calculate assignment sequences, we identified successive months when an individual's duty location changed. For each location, we computed the percentages of assignments originating from all other locations. Figure A.1 shows the percentages for the top five locations preceding WestPac assignments for 4N0X1.

Figure A.1. Assignment Flows into the Western Pacific for Career Field 4N0X1

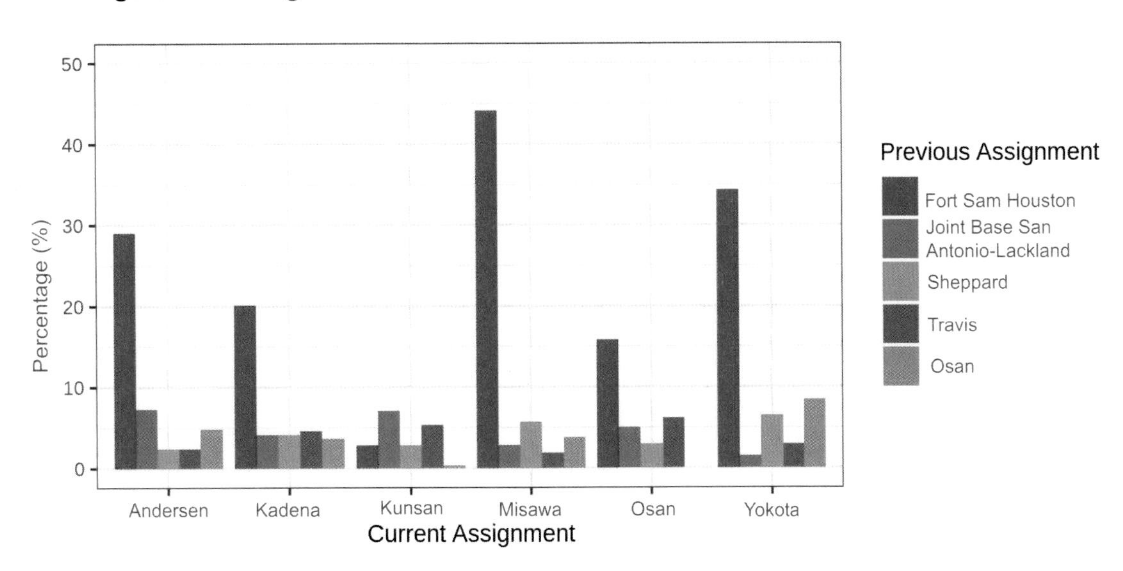

To calculate monthly assignment probabilities, we used a supervised machine learning approach called a generalized boosted model implemented in the R programming language. Based on historical data, the approach learns a sequence of decision rules to predict whether individuals will be reassigned in each month based on their AFSCs, locations, and TOS. Figure A.2 shows these probabilities for six WestPac locations for 4N0X1 assignments. The observed cumulative retention probabilities drop to around 12 months for Osan Air Base and Kunsan Air Base, two short-tour locations (top panel). The observed probabilities show a step-like shape for the other locations, reflecting the mixture of accompanied and unaccompanied tours for individuals at those locations. The statistical model of assignment probabilities also differentiated between short-tour locations and other locations (bottom panel).

To calculate monthly separation probabilities, we again used generalized boosted models to predict whether individuals will separate in each month based on their AFSCs, locations, TOS, and YOS. Figure A.3 shows the cumulative continuation rates (CCRs) formed after aggregating

Figure A.2. Cumulative Probability That an Individual Is Retained in an Existing Assignment over Time, by Western Pacific Location

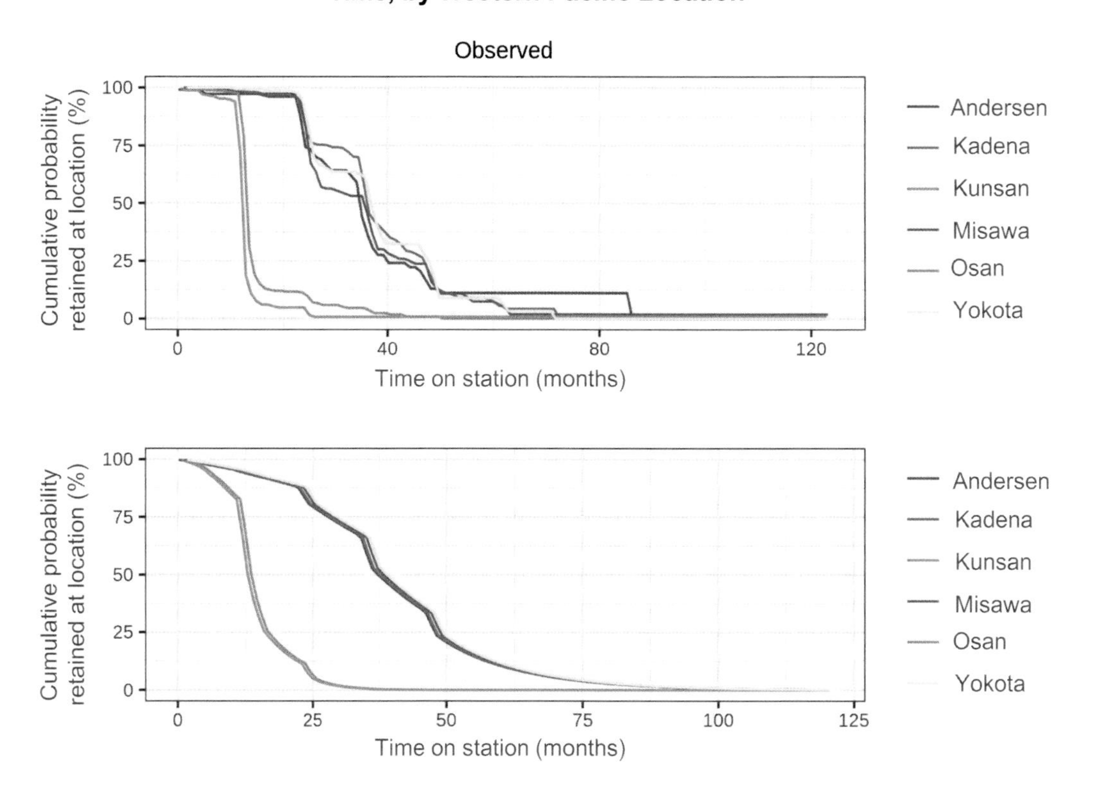

Figure A.3. Cumulative Continuation Rates for Career Field 4N0X1

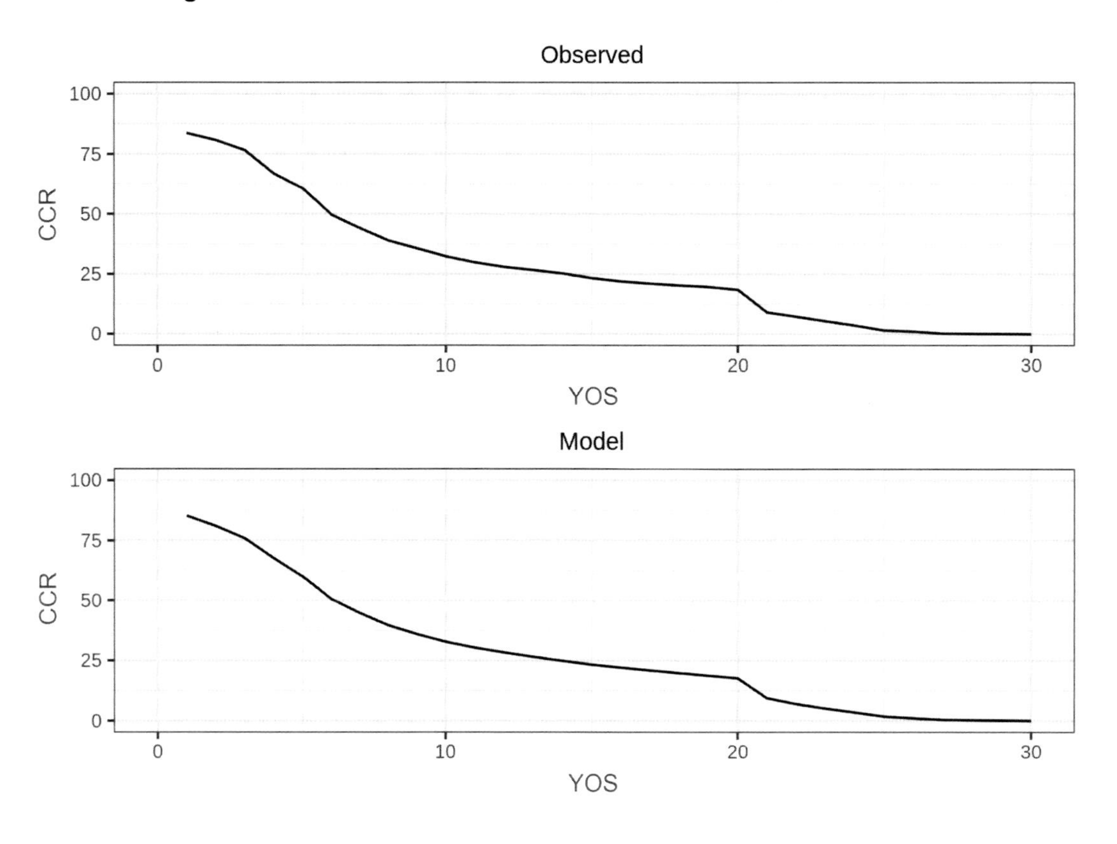

across location and TOS. The observed CCRs begin below 100 percent, reflecting the percentage of individuals who separated prior to completing initial skills training (top panel). The CCRs drop at a slightly accelerated rate during the fourth and sixth YOS, reflecting the conclusion of some individuals' four- and six-year initial service commitments. The CCRs plateau across midcareer values and drop again after 20 YOS as individuals retire. The statistical model re-creates the observed CCRs (bottom panel).

Parameters in the Computational Cognitive Model

The computational cognitive model contains two parameters corresponding to the rate of skill acquisition and the rate of skill decay. For the simulations reported in Chapter 4, the skill acquisition parameter was set to 0.05 (representing a relatively high rate of learning), and the skill decay parameter equaled 0.01 (a relatively lower rate of skill loss).[1] To test the sensitivity of the simulation to these parameters, we repeated the simulation three more times in order to compare model results for all four pairwise combinations of these values for the rate of skill acquisition and the rate of skill decay. Figures A.4–A.7 show average proficiency for all simulated critical AFSCs at WestPac locations. Tiles with dark borders denote the largest increase in proficiency relative to the baseline among simulations with one additional assignment policy (the second through fourth columns) and with two additional assignment policies (the fifth through seventh columns). The rank orderings of policy options were similar for different parameter values, with the exception that the benefits of reduced assignment duration were even greater when the rate of skill decay was high.

[1] Skill decay is often described in terms of half-life, or the time required for it to be reduced to half of its initial value. Likewise, skill acquisition can be described in terms of the time required to reduce the remaining mastery gap to half of its initial value. The values 0.05 and 0.01 correspond to a half-life of six and 24 months, respectively.

Figure A.4. Average Proficiency of Individuals in the Western Pacific by Air Force Specialty Code and Simulation for Model with High Learning Rate and Low Decay Rate

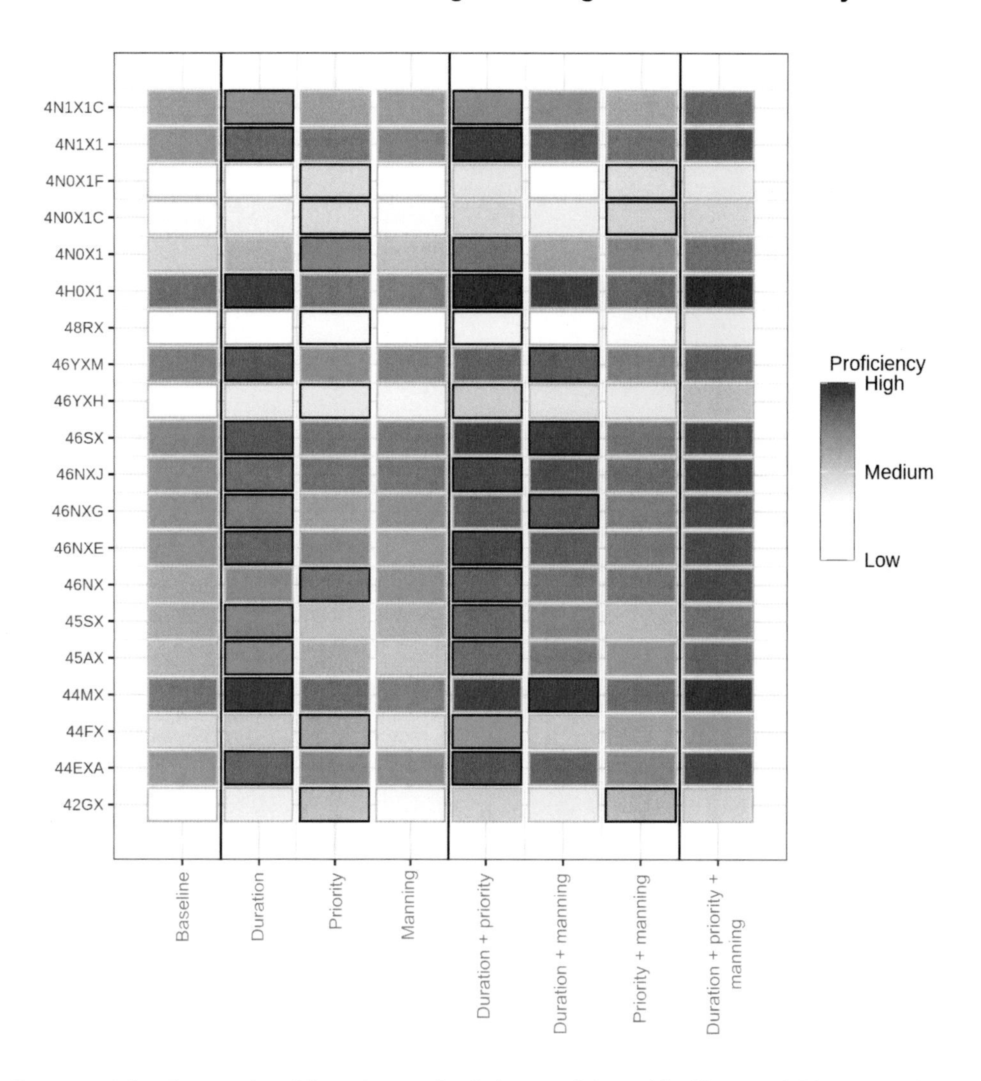

NOTE: This figure contains the results of the primary simulation model used in Chapter 4. These results are the same as those reported in Figure 4.4.

Figure A.5. Average Proficiency of Individuals in the Western Pacific by Air Force Specialty Code and Simulation for Model with High Learning Rate and High Decay Rate

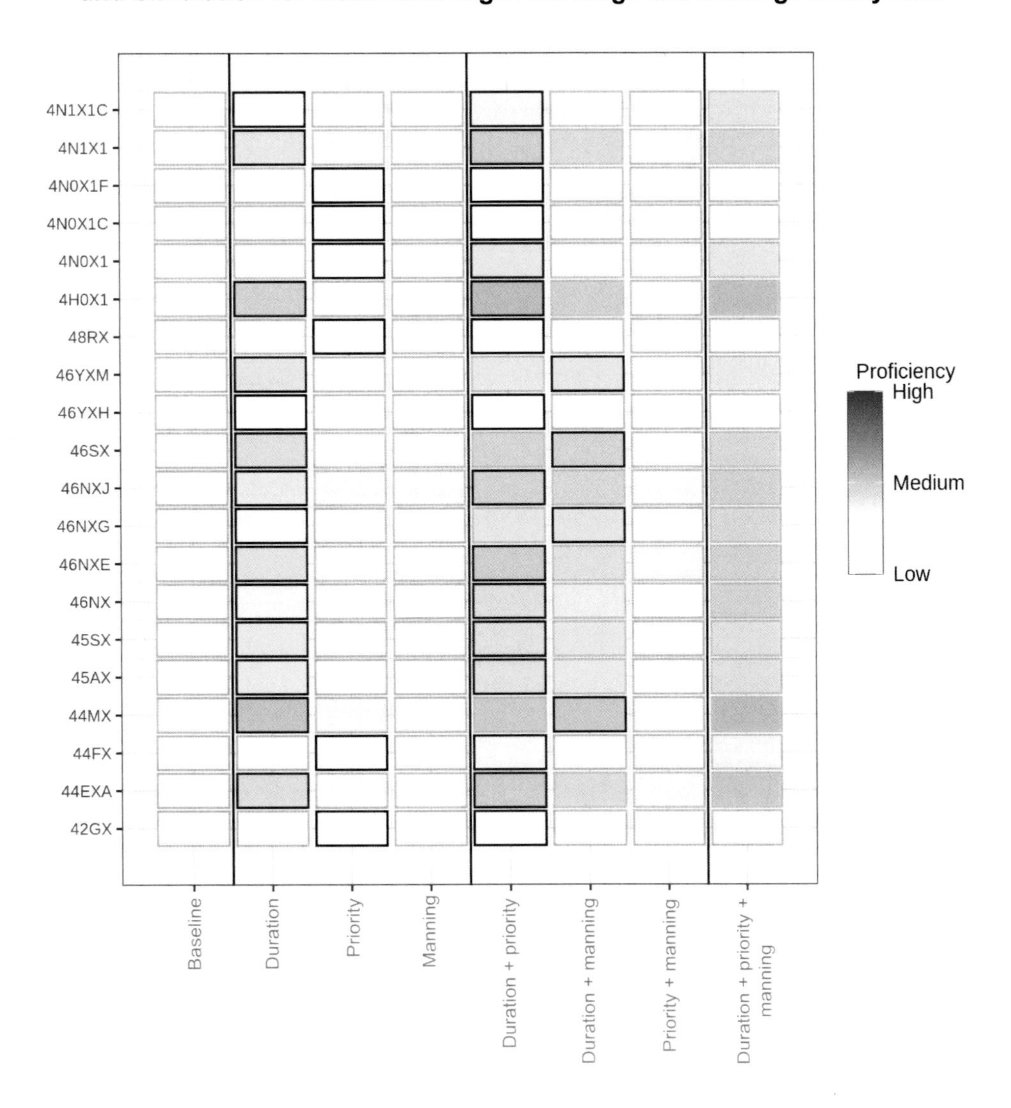

Figure A.6. Average Proficiency of Individuals in the Western Pacific by Air Force Specialty Code and Simulation for Model with Low Learning Rate and Low Decay Rate

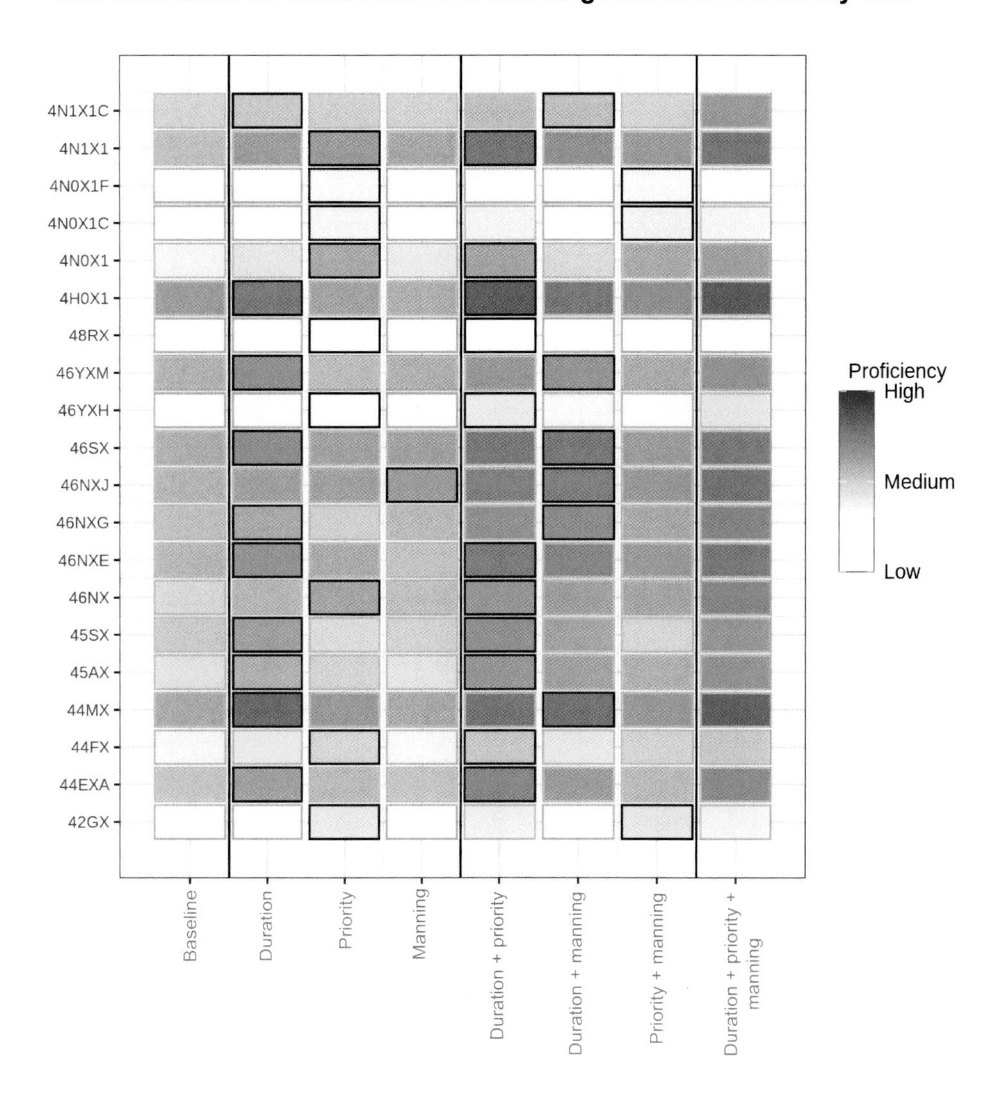

Figure A.7. Average Proficiency of Individuals in the Western Pacific by Air Force Specialty Code and Simulation for Model with Low Learning Rate and High Decay Rate

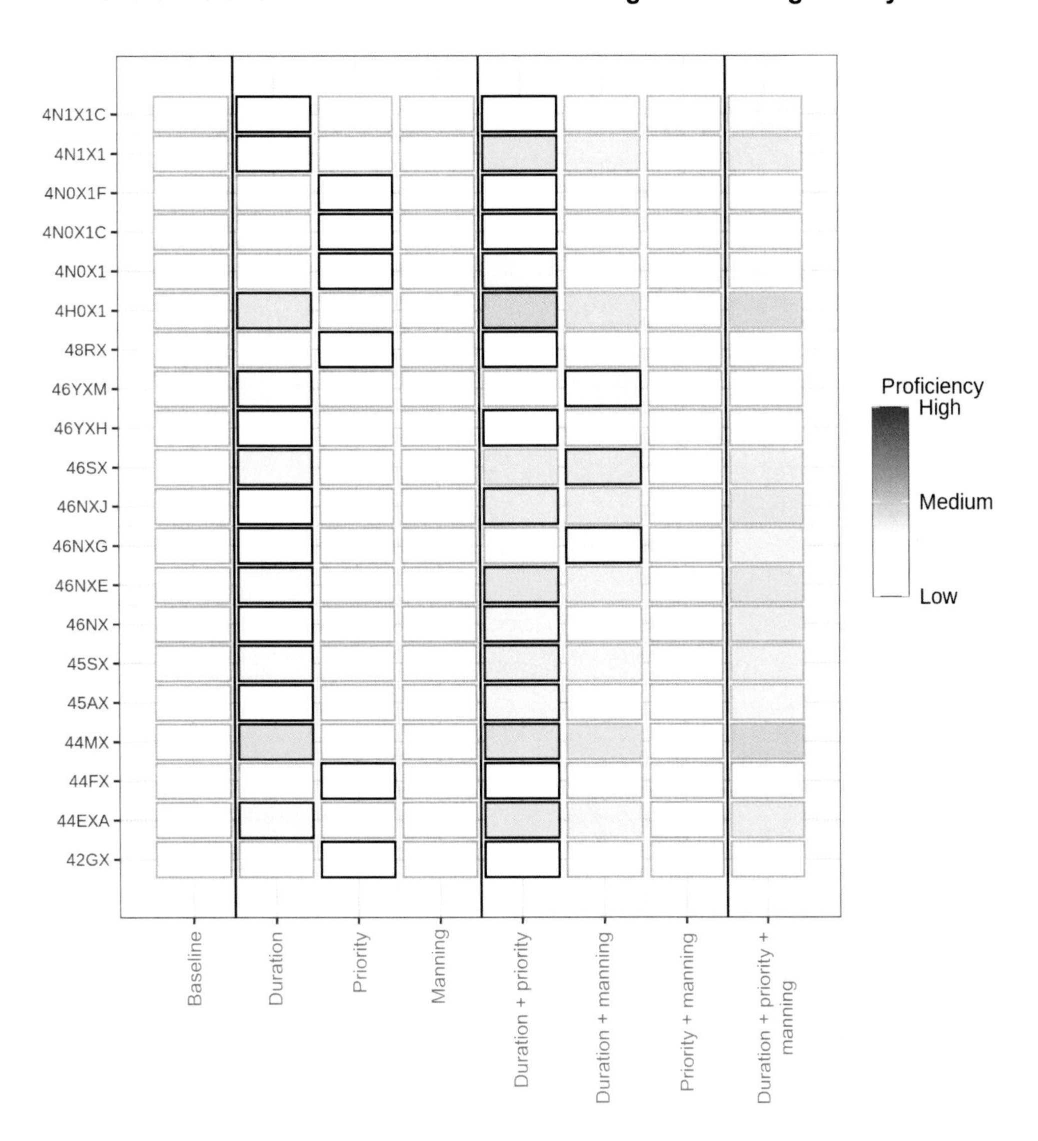

Appendix B. Reported Cost of Simulation Options

As was discussed in Chapter 3, expanding access to simulation training technology is one readiness building activity that could be used to improve clinical currency and readiness of medical personnel. The Air Force will need to make investments to expand such access, but identifying the right investments can be a challenge given the wide variety of simulation training options and the varied reported costs, examples of which are detailed in Table B.1.

Table B.1. Reported Costs of Simulation Options

Mode	Specific Intervention	Cost	Source
Training models	Burn escharotomy model	$1,152 for commercially available simulation kit; $75 to develop low-fidelity simulation model used in combination with free instructional video	Zhang, Thomas, Stewart, Curtis, Blayney, Mandell, Sohn, and Pham, 2020
	Emergency department thoracotomy model	$14,500 for commercially available model; $337 for custom model using commercially available clothes mannequin	Bengiamin, Toomasian, Smith, and Young, 2019
	Extracorporeal membrane oxygenation/CPR model	A$26,000 (~US$18,630) for commercially available extracorporeal membrane oxygenation model without airway or CPR functionality; A$4,625 (~US$3,300) to develop custom model, including A$2,025 (~US$1,450) for three-dimensional printed extracorporeal membrane oxygenation component and A$2,600 (~US$1,863) for CPR mannequin	Pang, Futter, Pincus, Dhanani, and Laupland, 2020
Courses	Three-day module for common emergency patient care scenarios in trauma and critical care surgery	$14,800 cost for three-day module or $2,960 per trained resident for simulated patient encounters using standardized patients and electronic mannequins to teach trauma and critical care skills	Miyasaka, Martin, Pascual, Buchholz, and Aggarwal, 2015[a]
	Otolaryngology “boot camp” for otolaryngology and emergency medicine residents	$16,000 for one-day “boot camp” with six cadaveric task trainer stations and four simulations	Cervenka, Hsieh, Sharon, and Bewley, 2020
	Adult life support course for primary care physicians and nurses	€29,034 (~US$33,150) per course or €1,320 (~US$1,500) per passed student for course with advanced simulator mannequins; €7,689 (~US$8,800) per course or €392 (~US$450) per passed student for course with standard mannequins	Iglesias-Vázquez, Rodríguez-Núñez, Penas-Penas, Sánchez-Santos, Cegarra-García, and Barreiro-Díaz, 2007[b]
	Obstetric emergency training course for doctors, midwives, and support workers in a hospital maternity unit	€148,806 (~US$170,000) to establish and run training, including €5,574 (~US$6,365) startup cost and €143,232 (~US$163,560) variable cost per year	Yau, Pizzo, Morris, Odd, Winter, and Draycott, 2016

Mode	Specific Intervention	Cost	Source
	Delivery of the Surgery Resident Skills Curriculum of the American College of Surgeons/Association of Program Directors in Surgery	$4 million setup cost, $22,000–$30,000 per year for staffing and faculty time, and $12,500–$33,000 per resident for simulation-based training to teach basic skills and tasks, advanced procedures, and team-based skills to general surgery residents	Stefanidis, Sevdalis, Paige, Zevin, Aggarwal, Grantcharov, and Jones, 2015[c]
Training centers	Simulation center	$876,485 setup cost, $361,425 fixed cost per year, $311 variable cost per course hour	McIntosh, Macario, Flanagan, and Gaba, 2006[d]
	Penn Medicine Clinical Simulation Center	$3.8 million capital cost, including physical plant, simulators, and advanced audiovisual system; $1.5 million total operating cost per year; $75 cost per participant for average group size of 18	Acero, Motuk, Luba, Murphy, McKelvey, Kolb, Dumon, and Resnick, 2012[e]
VR	High-end VR software	Approximately £3,000 (~US$4,050) for setup, including laptop and headset; software costs depend on provider and product quality, but frequently under one-tenth of the cost of physical simulation	Pottle, 2019
	Multiple VR trainers	$2,000–$100,000 or more	Hoopes, Pham, Lindo, and Antosh, 2020
	Low-cost flight simulator	$40,000–$45,000 for VR headset and stick and pedals with force feedback, compared with $26 million for traditional simulator	Hunter, 2021

[a] Kiyoyuki W. Miyasaka, Niels D. Martin, Jose L. Pascual, Joseph Buchholz, and Rajesh Aggarwal, "A Simulation Curriculum for Management of Trauma and Surgical Critical Care Patients," *Journal of Surgical Education*, Vol. 72, No. 5, September 2015.
[b] José Antonio Iglesias-Vázquez, Antonio Rodríguez-Núñez, Mónica Penas-Penas, Luís Sánchez-Santos, Maria Cegarra-García, and Maria Victoria Barreiro-Díaz, "Cost-Efficiency Assessment of Advanced Life Support (ALS) Courses Based on the Comparison of Advanced Simulators with Conventional Manikins," *BMC Emergency Medicine*, Vol. 7, No. 1, December 2007.
[c] Dimitrios Stefanidis, Nick Sevdalis, John Paige, Boris Zevin, Rajesh Aggarwal, Teodor Grantcharov, and Daniel B. Jones, "Simulation in Surgery: What's Needed Next?" *Annals of Surgery*, Vol. 261, No. 5, May 2015.
[d] Cate McIntosh, Alex Macario, Brendan Flanagan, and David Gaba, "Simulation: What Does It Really Cost?" *Simulation in Healthcare: Journal of the Society for Simulation in Healthcare*, Vol. 1, No. 2, 2006.
[e] Natalia Martinez Acero, Gregory Motuk, Josef Luba, Michael Murphy, Susan McKelvey, Gretchen Kolb, Kristoffel R. Dumon, and Andrew S. Resnick, "Managing a Surgical Exsanguination Emergency in the Operating Room Through Simulation: An Interdisciplinary Approach," *Journal of Surgical Education*, Vol. 69, No. 6, November 2012.

Appendix C. A Logic Model for Air Force Medical Service Medical Personnel Currency and Readiness

We constructed a logic model that illustrates how people, facilities, and programs combine to produce medical personnel who are ready for their wartime missions. A *logic model* describes visually the connection between the planned work of a program and the program's intended results. It includes *inputs*, the human, financial, and organizational resources available to the program; *activities*, the processes that make use of the inputs; *outputs*, the direct products of the activities; and *outcomes*, "specific changes in program participants' behavior, knowledge, skills, status and level of functioning."[1]

Logic models help build a common understanding of a program, identify critical factors—including partners, resources, links between organizational units and projects, and intermediate results—that could affect the outcome and identify measurement points and evaluation issues.[2] The Office of Management and Budget has encouraged federal agencies to include logic models in their evaluation plans.[3] RAND teams have used logical models to assist multiple federal agencies, including the Department of Homeland Security, DoD, the Federal Voting Assistance Program, the National Center for Injury Prevention and Control, and the National Institute for Occupational Safety and Health.[4]

Because the logic model depicted in Figure C.1 is primarily intended to be an example of the analysis the AFMS could do, the project team purposely built a simple model with enough elements to capture the distinguishing characteristics of the readiness building activities and policies discussed but without attempting to include every detail. Adjustments to this logic

---

[1] W. K. Kellogg Foundation, *Logic Model Development Guide*, January 2004.

[2] Sharon Caudle, "Homeland Security: Approaches to Results Management," *Public Performance and Management Review*, Vol. 28, No. 3, March 2005.

[3] Russell T. Vought, "Phase 1 Implementation of the Foundations for Evidence-Based Policymaking Act of 2018: Learning Agendas, Personnel, and Planning Guidance," Memorandum M-19-23, July 10, 2019.

[4] Christopher Paul, Brian J. Gordon, Jennifer D. P. Moroney, Lisa Saum-Manning, Beth Grill, Colin P. Clarke, and Heather Peterson, *A Building Partner Capacity Assessment Framework: Tracking Inputs, Outputs, Outcomes, Disrupters, and Workarounds*, RAND Corporation, RR-935-OSD, 2015; Victoria A. Greenfield, Henry H. Willis, and Tom LaTourrette, *Assessing the Benefits of U.S. Customs and Border Protection Regulatory Actions to Reduce Terrorism Risks*, RAND Corporation, CF-301-INDEC, 2012; Eric Landree, Hirokazu Miyake, and Victoria A. Greenfield, *Nanomaterial Safety in the Workplace: Pilot Project for Assessing the Impact of the NIOSH Nanotechnology Research Center*, RAND Corporation, RR-1108-NIOSH, 2015; Victoria A. Greenfield, Valerie L. Williams, and Elisa Eiseman, *Using Logic Models for Strategic Planning and Evaluation: Application to the National Center for Injury Prevention and Control*, RAND Corporation, TR-370-NCIPC, 2006; Victoria A. Greenfield, Shoshana R. Shelton, and Edward Balkovich, *The Role of Logic Modeling in a Collaborative and Iterative Research Process*, RAND Corporation, RR-882/1-OSD.

model could affect appropriate considerations for selecting and resourcing readiness building activities and policies.

Inputs

The inputs fall into six categories:

1. *AFMS personnel.* These are the personnel who are required to be current and ready, and they fall into two broad groups: (1) AFMS personnel assigned to WestPac, who must be prepared for the potential to "fight tonight"; and (2) PACAF personnel in Alaska and Hawaii or AFMS personnel in CONUS, who must be prepared to deploy to augment the forward-assigned WestPac personnel. A more detailed logic model could list out each AFSC or specialty.
2. *Cadres and trainers.* These are the personnel conducting the training—including, for example, the cadres based at C-STARS locations responsible for guiding students who attend the programs.
3. *Facilities.* In our model we focus on health care facilities. For most AFMS personnel, this would be MTFs, but it could also be civilian Level 1 trauma centers or VA hospitals, to name two possible types of partners.
4. *Patients.* Caring for patients is how medical personnel develop and maintain their skills. We divide patients into trauma, high-acuity nontrauma (i.e., critical care medicine), and those who are of relatively lower acuity.
5. *Time Commitment.* We use the term *hours* to indicate the amount of time spent on an activity. Time is captured to distinguish between readiness building activities that are full-time (e.g., embedding in a partner institution), part-time (e.g., intermittent work), or undertaken outside duty hours (e.g., ODE).
6. *Resources for TDY assignments and other overhead expenses.* Some readiness building activities require the student to travel. Other activities require the trainer to travel. There may also be other expenses related to establishing or maintaining programs. While the primary cost of most activities will be the time of the personnel involved, we wanted to recognize other related costs.

Figure C.1. The Logic Model for Air Force Medical Service Personnel Currency and Readiness

Inputs

AFMS personnel
- WestPac
- Alaska and Hawaii
- CONUS

Cadre and trainers

Facilities
- MTF
- Civilian Level 1 trauma centers
- VA medical centers

Patients
- Trauma
- High-acuity nontrauma
- Low-acuity

Time Commitment
- On-duty full-time
- On-duty part-time
- Off-duty

Resources for TDY and other overhead expenses

Activities

Practice
- Trauma
- High-acuity nontrauma
- Low-acuity

Training
- Observing care of trauma
- Classroom instruction
- Simulation and exercise

Personnel Management
- Workforce management
- Career development, including assignment actions

Outputs

Clinical hours worked
- Trauma
- High-acuity nontrauma
- Low-acuity

Courses attended

Simulations, exercises attended

Skills obtained
- CMRP
  - Currency
  - Readiness
- KSA

Outcomes

WestPac personnel ready to provide trauma care and critical care

CONUS, and Alaska and Hawaii, personnel ready to provide trauma care and critical care

Activities

The logic model activities reflect the readiness building activities and policies presented in Chapters 4 and 5. The first item, "Practice," is concerned with providing care to patients—the essence of the practice of medicine.[5] The type of care provided may be trauma, high-acuity nontrauma, or low-acuity care. Categories of training activities include rotations where students go on rounds; observing the care of trauma patients but not actually taking charge of patients themselves; as well as classroom instruction, online courses, medical simulations, and exercises. The personnel management policies in the logic model recognize that there are workforce decisions to be made, such as whether to assign uniformed or civilian personnel to certain positions or how to develop personnel in medical specialties over the course of a career.

Outputs

The model contains four observable and measurable outputs:

1. *Clinical hours worked.* The amount of time spent caring for patients of various types is the most immediate measure of the extent to which an Air Force clinician is actively practicing medicine. Alternatively, one could measure the number of patients seen or, for some specialties, the number and type of procedures performed. Capturing this data might be difficult, especially if electronic health records are not available; it may be easier to simply capture hours worked.
2. *Courses attended.* This output includes the number, type, and frequency of course attendance for Air Force personnel. Recording the classes and training events attended should be straightforward.
3. *Simulations and exercises attended.* Similarly, it should be straightforward to record and track participation in medical simulations and exercises.
4. *Skills obtained.* This output includes basic medical skills and wartime-specific skills for each specialty. These outputs are, to varying extents, tracked in two existing readiness measurement systems, CMRP/MDRSS and KSAs. As the KSA metric and reporting system becomes more developed, it can be added to the CMRP as an additional source of readiness information (as has already been done for General Surgery, 45SX).

Outcomes

The desired outcomes are the production of ready medical personnel in WestPac and throughout the AFMS.

---

[5] Wendy Levinson and Arthur Rubenstein, "Mission Critical—Integrating Clinician-Educators into Academic Medical Centers," *New England Journal of Medicine*, Vol. 341, No. 11, September 9, 1999.

Examples

We use two examples to illustrate the how the logic model is consistent with the readiness building activities and policies suggested by AFMS stakeholders and described in Chapter 3.

Example 1: Mandating Training at C-STARS Before or During PACAF Assignment. This readiness building activity can be traced using the logic model framework as follows. Inputs include personnel attending C-STARS either shortly before transferring to WestPac or at some point during their assignment to the region. Other inputs to the C-STARS activity include cadre members assigned to the program, as well as an established relationship with a civilian Level 1 trauma center, which provides the facilities and trauma patients that also serve as logic model inputs. The final inputs are the on-duty part-time hours that participants spend in the program and the TDY costs associated with their participation and travel.

At C-STARS, participants are involved in a combination of activities including classroom instruction, observation of trauma patients, and some direct involvement in the caring of trauma patients. The outputs of these activities include clinical hours spent caring for patients, as well as specific coursework and simulations attended, all of which could be recorded in the CMRP and MRDSS readiness measurement systems. The ultimate outcome of this completing this activity would be participants who more ready to provide effective care for trauma patients as needed in their upcoming or ongoing assignment to WestPac.

Example 2: Embedding at a VAMC. In this readiness building activity, the inputs include U.S.-based AFMS personnel assigned to be embedded, the VAMC hospitals that would host them, and the high-acuity nontrauma patients seen at those VAMCs. In cases where AFMS personnel are embedding at a VAMC as a cadre, they would further serve as cadre members in support of other Air Force medical providers providing care on a rotational or part-time basis. The time commitment input for AFMS personnel embedding at a VAMC (whether as a cadre or fully dedicated to patient care) would be full-time, though TDY dollars would not be a required input, as this would be a permanent military assignment.

In this example, the activity portion of the logic model framework would consist of participants caring for high-acuity nontrauma patients. The outputs of this activity would include the clinical hours spent providing such care, as well as the skills obtained and tracked using the CMRP or KSA readiness reporting systems. The outcome would be AFMS personnel who are ready to provide effective care for trauma patients in their next assignment to a WestPac, Hawaii, Alaska, CONUS, or OCONUS location.

Abbreviations

AFMS	Air Force Medical Service
AFPC	Air Force Personnel Center
AFSC	Air Force Specialty Code
CCR	cumulative continuation rate
CMRP	Comprehensive Medical Readiness Program
CONUS	continental United States
CPR	cardiopulmonary resuscitation
C-STARS	Center for the Sustainment of Trauma and Readiness Skills
CY	calendar year
DAF	Department of the Air Force
DHA	Defense Health Agency
DoD	Department of Defense
FTE	full-time equivalent
FY	fiscal year
IDMT	Independent Duty Medical Technician
KSA	knowledge, skills, and abilities
MAJCOM	major command
MHS	Military Health System
MOU	memorandum of understanding
MRDSS	Medical Resource Decision Support System
MTF	military treatment facility
NCO	noncommissioned officer
OCONUS	outside the continental United States
ODE	off-duty employment
PACAF	Pacific Air Forces
PAF	Project AIR FORCE
SMART	Sustained Medical and Readiness Trained

TAA	Training Affiliation Agreement
TDY	temporary duty
TOS	time on station
USAFSAM	U.S. Air Force School of Aerospace Medicine
VA	Veterans Affairs
VAMC	Veterans Affairs Medical Center
VR	virtual reality
WestPac	Western Pacific
YOS	years of service

Bibliography

Acero, Natalia Martinez, Gregory Motuk, Josef Luba, Michael Murphy, Susan McKelvey, Gretchen Kolb, Kristoffel R. Dumon, and Andrew S. Resnick, "Managing a Surgical Exsanguination Emergency in the Operating Room Through Simulation: An Interdisciplinary Approach," *Journal of Surgical Education*, Vol. 69, No. 6, November 2012, pp. 759–765.

AFPC—*See* Air Force Personnel Center.

Ahlberg, Gunnar, Lars Enochsson, Anthony G. Gallagher, Leif Hedman, Christian Hogman, David A. McClusky III, Stig Ramel, C. Daniel Smith, and Dag Arvidsson, "Proficiency-Based Virtual Reality Training Significantly Reduces the Error Rate for Residents During Their First 10 Laparoscopic Cholecystectomies," *American Journal of Surgery*, Vol. 193, No. 6, June 2007, pp. 797–804.

Air Force Instruction 36-2110, *Total Force Assignments*, Department of the Air Force, November 15, 2021. As of January 8, 2023: https://static.e-publishing.af.mil/production/1/af_a1/publication/dafi36-2110/dafi36-2110.pdf

Air Force Instruction 41-106, *Air Force Medical Readiness Program*, Department of the Air Force, July 29, 2020. As of January 8, 2023: https://static.e-publishing.af.mil/production/1/af_sg/publication/afi41-106/afi41-106.pdf

Air Force Instruction 44-102, *Medical Care Management*, Department of the Air Force, March 17, 2015. As of January 8, 2023: https://static.e-publishing.af.mil/production/1/af_sg/publication/afi44-102/afi44-102_afgm2022-01.pdf

Air Force Manual 41-108, *Training Affiliation Agreement Program*, Department of the Air Force, August 21, 2019. As of January 8, 2023: https://static.e-publishing.af.mil/production/1/af_sg/publication/afman41-108/afman41-108.pdf

Air Force Personnel Center, *Air Force Enlisted Classification Directory (AFECD): The Official Guide to the Air Force Enlisted Classification Codes*, April 30, 2021a.

Air Force Personnel Center, *Air Force Officer Classification Directory (AFOCD): The Official Guide to the Air Force Officer Classification Codes*, April 30, 2021b.

Alia-Novobilski, Marisa, "C-STARS Visit Highlights Trauma Training," Air Force Medical Service, June 19, 2018. As of September 7, 2021: https://www.airforcemedicine.af.mil/News/Display/Article/1553842/c-stars-visit-highlights-trauma-training/

American Association of Critical-Care Nurses, "Board Certification," webpage, undated. As of November 21, 2022:
https://www.aacn.org/certification

American College of Surgeons, *The Blue Book: Military-Civilian Partnerships for Trauma Training, Sustainment, and Readiness*, 2020.

American College of Surgeons, Committee on Trauma, *Resources for Optimal Care of the Injured Patient*, 2014. As of September 8, 2021:
https://www.facs.org/-/media/files/quality-programs/trauma/vrc-resources/resources-for-optimal-care.ashx

Anderson, John R., and Christian D. Schunn, "Implications of the ACT-R Learning Theory: No Magic Bullets," in Robert Glaser, ed., *Advances in Instructional Psychology*: Vol. 5, *Educational Design and Cognitive Science*, Lawrence Erlbaum Associates, Inc., 2000.

Arthur, Winfred, Jr., Winston Bennett Jr., Pamela L. Stanush, and Theresa L. McNelly, "Factors That Influence Skill Decay and Retention: A Quantitative Review and Analysis," *Human Performance*, Vol. 11, No. 1, 1998, pp. 57–101.

Auganix.org, "SimX Receives New U.S. Air Force Contracts Totaling over $1.5 Million to Advance Virtual Reality Training Programs," May 3, 2021. As of September 24, 2021:
https://www.auganix.org/simx-receives-new-us-air-force-contracts-totaling-over-1-5-million-to-advance-virtual-reality-training-programs/

Avila, Jaie, "Legislation Would Allow BAMC to Waive Big, Surprise Bills for Some Patients," News 4 San Antonio, December 18, 2020. As of September 7, 2021:
https://news4sanantonio.com/news/trouble-shooters/legislation-would-allow-bamc-to-waive-big-surprise-bills-for-some-patients

Bengiamin, Deena I., Cory Toomasian, Dustin D. Smith, and Timothy P. Young, "Emergency Department Thoracotomy: A Cost-Effective Model for Simulation Training," *Journal of Emergency Medicine*, Vol. 57, No. 3, September 2019, pp. 375–379.

Berwick, Donald, Autumn Downey, and Elizabeth Cornett, eds., *A National Trauma Care System: Integrating Military and Civilian Trauma Systems to Achieve Zero Preventable Deaths After Injury*, National Academies Press, 2016.

Broomfield, Rebecca, "A Quasi-Experimental Research to Investigate the Retention of Basic Cardiopulmonary Resuscitation Skills and Knowledge by Qualified Nurses Following a Course in Professional Development," *Journal of Advanced Nursing*, Vol. 23, No. 5, June 28, 2008, pp. 1016–1023.

Cannon, Jeremy W., Kirby R. Gross, and Todd E. Rasmussen, "Combating the Peacetime Effect in Military Medicine," *JAMA Surgery*, September 2020, pp. 5–6.

Carius, Brandon M., Michael D. April, and Steve G. Schauer, "Procedural Volume Within Military Treatment Facilities—Implications for a Ready Medical Force," *Military Medicine*, Vol. 185, Nos. 7–8, July–August 2020, pp. e977–e981.

Caudle, Sharon, "Homeland Security: Approaches to Results Management," *Public Performance and Management Review*, Vol. 28, No. 3, March 2005, pp. 352–375.

Cecilio-Fernandes, Dario, Fokie Cnossen, Debbie A. D. C. Jaarsma, and René A. Tio, "Avoiding Surgical Skill Decay: A Systematic Review on the Spacing of Training Sessions," *Journal of Surgical Education*, Vol. 75, No. 2, March 2018, pp. 471–480.

Cervenka, Brian P., Tsung-yen Hsieh, Sharon Lin, and Arnaud Bewley, "Multi-Institutional Regional Otolaryngology Bootcamp," *Annals of Otology, Rhinology and Laryngology*, Vol. 129, No. 6, June 2020, pp. 605–610.

Chan, Edward W., Heather Krull, Sangeeta C. Ahluwalia, James R. Broyles, Daniel A. Waxman, Jill Gurvey, Paul M. Colthirst, JoEllen Schimmels, and Anthony Marinos, *Options for Maintaining Clinical Proficiency During Peacetime*, RAND Corporation, RR-2543-A, 2020. As of September 5, 2021:
https://www.rand.org/pubs/research_reports/RR2543.html

Chen, Lena M., Marta Render, Anne Sales, Edward H. Kennedy, Wyndy Wiitala, and Timothy P. Hofer, "Intensive Care Unit Admitting Patterns in the Veterans Affairs Health Care System," *Archives of Internal Medicine*, Vol. 172, No. 16, September 2012, pp. 1220–1226.

Competency and Credentialing Institute, "Certified Perioperative Nurse," webpage, undated. As of September 5, 2021:
https://www.cc-institute.org/cnor/learn/

Cox, Daniel B., "Managing a Mature Military-Civilian Partnership: Civilian Perspective," UAB School of Medicine, briefing, undated. As of September 7, 2021:
https://www.amsus.org/wp-content/uploads/2019/12/Cox-AMSUS-Mil-Civ-partnership-2019.pdf

Davenport, Daniel L., William G. Henderson, Cecilia L. Mosca, Shukri F. Khuri, and Robert M. Mentzer, Jr., "Risk-Adjusted Morbidity in Teaching Hospitals Correlates with Reported Levels of Communication and Collaboration on Surgical Teams but Not with Scale Measures of Teamwork Climate, Safety Climate, or Working Conditions," *Journal of American College of Surgeons*, Vol. 205, No. 6, December 2007, pp. 778–784.

Davidson, Philip S., "U.S. Indo-Pacific Command Posture," statement before the Committee on Armed Services, U.S. Senate, March 9, 2021. As of September 5, 2021:
https://www.armed-services.senate.gov/imo/media/doc/Davidson_03-09-21.pdf

Deputy Group Commander Chief Nurse, "Sustained Medical & Readiness Trained (SMART)," 6th Medical Group, briefing, undated. As of September 7, 2021: https://www.health.mil/Reference-Center/Presentations/2015/11/09/Civilian-Partnerships-for-Training-Currency-and-Business-Plans-Develop-SMART

DoD—*See* U.S. Department of Defense.

Dougherty, Adam, "SimX Receives New U.S. Air Force Contracts to Advance VR Training Programs, Explore Space Warfighter Readiness," SimX, May 14, 2021. As of September 6, 2021: https://www.simxvr.com/blog/simx-receives-air-force-contracts/

Eastridge, Brian J., Robert L. Mabry, Peter Seguin, Joyce Cantrell, Terrill Tops, Paul Uribe, Olga Mallett, Tamara Zubko, Lynne Oetjen-Gerdes, Todd E. Rasmussen, Frank K. Butler, Russell S. Kotwal, John B. Holcomb, Charles Wade, Howard Champion, Mimi Lawnick, Leon Moores, and Lorne H. Blackbourne, "Death on the Battlefield (2001–2011): Implications for the Future of Combat Casualty Care," *Journal of Trauma and Acute Care Surgery*, Vol. 73, No. 6, December 2012, pp. S431–S437.

Ediger, Mark, "Air Force Medical Service: Focus Areas in Action," Headquarters U.S. Air Force, briefing, February 9, 2017. As of September 7, 2021: https://www.health.mil/Reference-Center/Presentations/2017/02/09/Overview-of-Air-Force-Medical-Service

Eubanks, Allison A., Keith Volner, and Joseph O. Lopreiato, *Past Present and Future of Simulation in Military Medicine*, Treasure Island, Fla.: StatPearls Publishing, November 14, 2020. As of September 25, 2021: https://www.ncbi.nlm.nih.gov/books/NBK553172/

Farrell, Brenda S., *Military Personnel: Additional Actions Needed to Address Gaps in Military Physician Specialties*, U.S. Government Accountability Office, GAO-18-77, 2018.

Feldscher, Jacqueline, "China Is Our No. 1 Priority. Start Acting Like It, Austin Tells Pentagon," *Defense One*, June 9, 2021.

Fitzpatrick, Kevin F., and Paul F. Pasquina, "Overview of the Rehabilitation of the Combat Casualty," *Military Medicine*, Vol. 175, No. 7S, July 2010, pp. 013–017.

Goldberg, Matthew S., "Comparing the Costs of the Veterans' Health Care System with Private-Sector Costs," testimony before the Subcommittee on Health, Committee on Veterans' Affairs, U.S. House of Representatives, Congressional Budget Office, January 28, 2015. As of September 7, 2021: http://www.cbo.gov/sites/default/files/cbofiles/attachments/49905-Testimony.pdf

Grantcharov, Teodor P., Viggo B. Kristiansen, Jørgen Bendix, Linda Bardram, Jacob Rosenberg, and Peter Funch-Jensen, "Randomized Clinical Trial of Virtual Reality Simulation for Laparoscopic Skills Training," *British Journal of Surgery*, Vol. 91, No. 2, February 2004, pp. 146–150.

Graser, John C., Daniel Blum, Kevin Brancato, James J. Burks, Edward W. Chan, Nancy Nicosia, Michael J. Neumann, Hans V. Ritschard, and Benjamin F. Mundell, *The Economics of Air Force Medical Service Readiness*, RAND Corporation, TR-859-AF, 2010. As of September 7, 2021:
https://www.rand.org/pubs/technical_reports/TR859.html

Greenfield, Victoria A., Shoshana R. Shelton, and Edward Balkovich, *The Role of Logic Modeling in a Collaborative and Iterative Research Process*, RAND Corporation, RR-882/1-OSD. As of September 10, 2021:
https://www.rand.org/pubs/research_reports/RR882z1.html

Greenfield, Victoria A., Valerie L. Williams, and Elisa Eiseman, *Using Logic Models for Strategic Planning and Evaluation: Application to the National Center for Injury Prevention and Control*, RAND Corporation, TR-370-NCIPC, 2006. As of September 10, 2021:
http://www.rand.org/pubs/technical_reports/TR370.html

Greenfield, Victoria A., Henry H. Willis, and Tom LaTourrette, *Assessing the Benefits of U.S. Customs and Border Protection Regulatory Actions to Reduce Terrorism Risks*, RAND Corporation, CF-301-INDEC, 2012. As of September 10, 2021:
https://www.rand.org/pubs/conf_proceedings/CF301.html

Health.mil, "Patient Care Numbers for the Military Health System," webpage, undated-a. As of January 7, 2023:
https://health.mil/Military-Health-Topics/MHS-Toolkits/Media-Resources/Media-Center/Patient-Care-Numbers-for-the-MHS

Health.mil, "Patients by TRICARE Plan," webpage, undated-b. As of January 7, 2023:
https://health.mil/Military-Health-Topics/MHS-Toolkits/Media-Resources/Media-Center/Patient-Population-Statistics/Patients-by-TRICARE-Plan

Higgins, Mark, Christopher Madan, and Rakesh Patel, "Development and Decay of Procedural Skills in Surgery: A Systematic Review of the Effectiveness of Simulation-Based Medical Education Interventions," *The Surgeon*, Vol. 19, No. 4, August 2021, pp. e67–e77.

Holt, Danielle B., Matthew T. Hueman, Jonathan Jaffin, Michael Sanchez, Mark A. Hamilton, Charles D. Mabry, Jeffrey A. Bailey, and Eric A. Elster, "Clinical Readiness Program: Refocusing the Military Health System," *Military Medicine*, Vol. 186, No. 1, January 25, 2021, pp. 32–39.

Hoopes, Sarah, Truce Pham, Fiona M. Lindo, and Danielle D. Antosh, “Home Surgical Skill Training Resources for Obstetrics and Gynecology Trainees During a Pandemic,” *Obstetrics and Gynecology*, Vol. 136, No. 1, July 2020, pp. 56–64.

Hunter, Jamie, “The Truth About the Air Force’s Biggest Changes to Pilot Training Since the Dawn of the Jet Age,” *The Drive*, August 3, 2021. As of September 25, 2021: https://www.thedrive.com/the-war-zone/41789/the-truth-about-the-air-forces-biggest-changes-to-pilot-training-since-the-dawn-of-the-jet-age

Iglesias-Vázquez, José Antonio, Antonio Rodríguez-Núñez, Mónica Penas-Penas, Luís Sánchez-Santos, Maria Cegarra-García, and Maria Victoria Barreiro-Díaz, “Cost-Efficiency Assessment of Advanced Life Support (ALS) Courses Based on the Comparison of Advanced Simulators with Conventional Manikins,” *BMC Emergency Medicine*, Vol. 7, No. 1, December 2007, pp. 18–22.

Jaffee, Michael S., Kathy M. Helmick, Philip D. Girard, Kim S. Meyer, Kathy Dinegar, and Karyn George, “Acute Clinical Care and Care Coordination for Traumatic Brain Injury within Department of Defense,” *Journal of Rehabilitation Research and Development*, Vol. 46, No. 6, 2009, pp. 655–666.

Jastrzembski, Tiffany S., Matthew M. Walsh, Michael Krusmark, Suzan Kardong-Edgren, Marilyn H. Oermann, Karey Dufour, Teresa Millwater, Kevin Gluck, Glenn Gunzelmann, Jack Harris, and Dimitrios Stefanidis, “Personalizing Training to Acquire and Sustain Competence Through Use of a Cognitive Model,” in Dylan D. Schmorrow and Cali M. Fidopiastis, eds., *Augmented Cognition: Enhancing Cognition and Behavior in Complex Human Environments*, Springer, 2017, pp. 148–161.

Kellicut, Dwight C., Eric J. Kuncir, Hope M. Williamson, Pamela C. Masella, and Peter E. Nielsen, “Surgical Team Assessment Training: Improving Surgical Teams During Deployment,” *American Journal of Surgery*, Vol. 208, No. 2, May 2014, pp. 275–283.

Kime, Patricia, “Plans for Hospital Closures as Part of Military Health System Reform Forging Ahead After Pause,” Military.com, March 30, 2022. As of November 19, 2022: https://www.military.com/daily-news/2022/03/30/plans-hospital-closures-part-of-military-health-system-reform-forging-ahead-after-pause.html

Landree, Eric, Hirokazu Miyake, and Victoria A. Greenfield, *Nanomaterial Safety in the Workplace: Pilot Project for Assessing the Impact of the NIOSH Nanotechnology Research Center*, RAND Corporation, RR-1108-NIOSH, 2015. As of September 10, 2021: http://www.rand.org/pubs/research_reports/RR1108.html

Legoux, Camille, Richard Gerein, Kathy Boutis, Nicholas Barrowman, and Amy Plint, “Retention of Critical Procedural Skills After Simulation Training: A Systematic Review,” *AEM Education and Training*, Vol. 5, No. 3, July 2021, article e10536.

Levinson, Wendy, and Arthur Rubenstein, "Mission Critical—Integrating Clinician-Educators into Academic Medical Centers," *New England Journal of Medicine*, Vol. 341, No. 11, September 9, 1999, pp. 840–843.

Lohre, Ryan, Jeffrey C. Wang, Kai-Uwe Lewandrowski, and Danny P. Goel, "Virtual Reality in Spinal Endoscopy: A Paradigm Shift in Education to Support Spine Surgeons," *Journal of Spine Surgery*, Vol. 6, No. S1, January 2020, pp. S208–S223.

Madden, Catherine, "Undergraduate Nursing Students' Acquisition and Retention of CPR Knowledge and Skills," *Nurse Education Today*, Vol. 26, No. 3, April 2006, pp. 218–227.

Martinez, Jodi, "C-STARS Sets New DoD Training Standard with New Simulator," U. S. Air Force, March 8, 2017. As of September 7, 2021: https://www.af.mil/News/Article-Display/Article/1106423/c-stars-sets-new-dod-training -standard-with-new-simulator/

Masserly, Megan, and Jackie Valley, "Heated Topic in Health Care: Does Las Vegas Have Enough Trauma Centers?" *Las Vegas Sun*, April 7, 2016. As of September 8, 2021: https://lasvegassun.com/news/2016/apr/07/heated-topic-in-health-care-does-las-vegas -have-en/

Mazzocco, Karen, Diana B. Petitti, Kenneth T. Fong, Doug Bonacum, John Brookey, Suzanne Graham, Robert E. Lasky, J. Bryan Sexton, and Eric J. Thomas, "Surgical Team Behaviors and Patient Outcomes," *American Journal of Surgery*, Vol. 197, No. 5, May 2009, pp. 678–685.

McIntosh, Cate, Alex Macario, Brendan Flanagan, and David Gaba, "Simulation: What Does It Really Cost?" *Simulation in Healthcare: Journal of the Society for Simulation in Healthcare*, Vol. 1, No. 2, 2006, p. 109.

Meiners, Martin, "JBSA–Fort Sam Houston Experts Provide Fort Campbell Medics Brigade Combat Team Trauma Training," Joint Base San Antonio, March 21, 2017. As of September 7, 2021: https://www.jbsa.mil/News/News/Article/1124912/jbsa-fort-sam-houston-experts-provide -fort-campbell-medics-brigade-combat-team/

MHS—*See* Military Health System.

Military Health System, *Military Health System Modernization Study Team Report*, Office of the Under Secretary of Defense for Personnel and Readiness, May 29, 2015.

Miyasaka, Kiyoyuki W., Niels D. Martin, Jose L. Pascual, Joseph Buchholz, and Rajesh Aggarwal, "A Simulation Curriculum for Management of Trauma and Surgical Critical Care Patients," *Journal of Surgical Education*, Vol. 72, No. 5, September 2015, pp. 803–810.

Mosley, C. M. J., and B. N. J. Shaw, "A Longitudinal Cohort Study to Investigate the Retention of Knowledge and Skills Following Attendance on the Newborn Life Support Course," *Archives of Disease in Childhood*, Vol. 98, No. 8, August 1, 2013, pp. 582–586.

Moulton, Carol-Anne E., Adam Dubrowski, Helen MacRae, Brent Graham, Ethan Grober, and Richard Reznick, "Teaching Surgical Skills: What Kind of Practice Makes Perfect? A Randomized, Controlled Trial," *Annals of Surgery*, Vol. 244, No. 3, 2006, pp. 400–409.

Naval Medical Center Camp Lejeune, "Trauma Center," webpage, undated. As of September 7, 2021:
https://camp-lejeune.tricare.mil/Health-Services/Urgent-Emergency-Care/Trauma-Center

Nelson, Kathleen, "SSM Health Hospital Trains Military Medical Personnel Headed to Combat Zones," Catholic Health Association of the United States, April 15, 2018. As of November 19, 2022:
https://www.chausa.org/publications/catholic-health-world/article/april-15-2018/ssm-health-hospital-trains-military-medical-personnel-headed-to-combat-zones

Oprihory, Jennifer-Leigh, "USAF Brings Pilot Training Next to Regular Training in Experimental Curriculum," *Air and Space Forces Magazine*, March 12, 2020. As of September 25, 2021:
https://www.airforcemag.com/usaf-brings-pilot-training-next-to-regular-training-in-experimental-curriculum/

O'Rourke, Ronald, *Renewed Great Power Competition: Implications for Defense—Issues for Congress*, Congressional Research Service, R43838, August 3, 2021.

PACAF—*See* Pacific Air Forces.

Pacific Air Forces, "Info," webpage, undated. As of September 4, 2021:
https://www.pacaf.af.mil/Info/

Pang, G., C. Futter, J. Pincus, J. Dhanani, and K. B. Laupland, "Development and Testing of a Low Cost Simulation Manikin for Extracorporeal Cardiopulmonary Resuscitation (ECPR) Using 3-Dimensional Printing," *Resuscitation*, Vol. 149, April 2020, pp. 24–29.

Paul, Christopher, Brian J. Gordon, Jennifer D. P. Moroney, Lisa Saum-Manning, Beth Grill, Colin P. Clarke, and Heather Peterson, *A Building Partner Capacity Assessment Framework: Tracking Inputs, Outputs, Outcomes, Disrupters, and Workarounds*, RAND Corporation, RR-935-OSD, 2015. As of September 10, 2021:
https://www.rand.org/pubs/research_reports/RR935.html

Perez, Ray S., Anna Skinner, Peter Weyhrauch, James Niehaus, Corinna Lathan, Steven D. Schwaitzberg, and Caroline G. L. Cao, "Prevention of Surgical Skill Decay," *Military Medicine*, Vol. 178, No. 10S, October 2013, pp. 76–86.

Pottle, Jack, "Virtual Reality and the Transformation of Medical Education," *Future Healthcare Journal*, Vol. 6, No. 3, October 2019, pp. 181–185.

RAND Corporation, *Assessment A (Demographics)*, September 1, 2015. As of November 19, 2022:
https://pdf4pro.com/view/assessment-a-demographics-292972.html

Reuters, "Remember: 'China, China, China,' New Acting U.S. Defense Secretary Says," January 2, 2019. As of November 19, 2022:
https://www.reuters.com/article/usa-military-china/remember-china-china-china-new-acting-u-s-defense-secretary-says-idUSL1N1Z20JA

Rhue, Alexandra L., and Beth VanDerveer, "Wilderness First Responder: Are Skills Soon Forgotten?" *Wilderness and Environmental Medicine*, Vol. 29, No. 1, March 2018, pp. 132–137.

Sall, Dana, Eric J. Warm, Benjamin Kinnear, Matthew Kelleher, Roman Jandarov, and Jennifer O'Toole, "See One, Do One, Forget One: Early Skill Decay After Paracentesis Training," *Journal of General Internal Medicine*, Vol. 36, No. 5, May 2021, pp. 1346–1351.

Sanchez, Elaine, "BAMC Takes On Additional Trauma Patients," U. S. Army, January 7, 2021. As of September 7, 2021:
https://www.army.mil/article/242231/bamc_takes_on_additional_trauma_patients

Smith, Kimberly K,. Darlene Gilcreast, and Karen Pierce, "Evaluation of Staff's Retention of ACLS and BLS Skills," *Resuscitation*, Vol. 78, No. 1, July 2008, pp. 59–65.

Stefanidis, Dimitrios, Nick Sevdalis, John Paige, Boris Zevin, Rajesh Aggarwal, Teodor Grantcharov, and Daniel B. Jones, "Simulation in Surgery: What's Needed Next?" *Annals of Surgery*, Vol. 261, No. 5, May 2015, pp. 846–853.

Thomas, Brent, *Preparing for the Future of Combat Casualty Care: Opportunities to Refine the Military Health System's Alignment with the National Defense Strategy*, Santa Monica, Calif.: RAND Corporation, RR-A713-1, 2021. As of September 7, 2021:
https://www.rand.org/pubs/research_reports/RRA713-1.html

Thorson, Chad M., Joseph J. Dubose, Peter Rhee, Thomas E. Knuth, Warren C. Dorlac, Jeffrey A. Bailey, George D. Garcia, Mark L. Ryan, Robert M. Van Haren, and Kenneth G. Proctor, "Military Trauma Training at Civilian Centers: A Decade of Advancements," *Journal of Trauma and Acute Care Surgery*, Vol. 73, No. 6, December 2012, pp. S483–S489.

TRICARE, "Types of Military Facilities," webpage, June 15, 2021. As of September 7, 2021:
https://tricare.mil/Military-Hospitals-and-Clinics/Types-of-Military-Facilities

UC Health, "C-STARS: University of Cincinnati Medical Center Cincinnati C-STARS," webpage, undated. As of September 7, 2021: https://www.uchealth.com/education/c-stars/

Uniformed Services University, "Clinical Readiness Program: Combat Casualty Care KSAs," briefing, April 2018. As of September 7, 2021: https://health.mil/Reference-Center/Presentations/2018/04/23/Combat-Casualty-Care-KSAs

University of Cincinnati Medical Center, "C-STARS Simulation Center Helps U.S. Air Force Medical Personnel Train," webpage, undated. As of September 7, 2021: https://www.uchealth.com/pulmonary-insights/simulation-center-helps-u-s-air-force-medical-personnel-train/

University of Maryland School of Medicine, "C-STARS (Center for the Sustainment of Trauma and Readiness Skills)," webpage, undated. As of September 7, 2021: https://www.medschool.umaryland.edu/trauma/education/c-stars-center-for-the-sustainment-of-trauma-and-readiness-skills/

U.S. Air Force, *USAF Strategic Master Plan*, May 2015. As of September 5, 2021: https://www.af.mil/Portals/1/documents/Force%20Management/Strategic_Master_Plan.pdf

U.S. Army Medical Department and School, U.S. Army Health Readiness Center of Excellence, *Course Catalog 2018*, Joint Base San Antonio, August 2017. As of August 18, 2021: https://ckapfwstor001.blob.core.usgovcloudapi.net/pfw-images/dbimages/AMEDDC&S%20Catalog%20FY18%20draft%20as%20of%2014%20SEPT%202017.pdf

U.S. Department of Defense, *Summary of the 2018 National Defense Strategy of the United States of America: Sharpening the American Military's Competitive Edge*, 2018.

U.S. Department of Defense, *Restructuring and Realignment of Military Medical Treatment Facilities: Report to the Congressional Defense Committees*, Office of the Under Secretary of Defense for Personnel and Readiness, February 19, 2020.

U.S. Department of Veterans Affairs, Veterans Health Administration, *2012 VHA Facility Quality and Safety Report*, September 2012. As of September 7, 2021: https://www.va.gov/health/docs/2012_vha_facility_quality_and_safety_report_final508.pdf

U.S. General Services Administration, "FY 2023 Per Diem Highlights," webpage, August 12, 2021. As of September 13, 2021: https://www.gsa.gov/travel/plan-book/per-diem-rates/fy-2022-per-diem-highlights

U.S. Government Accountability Office, *VA and DoD Health Care: Department-Level Actions Needed to Assess Collaboration Performance, Address Barriers, and Identify Opportunities*, GAO-12-992, September 2012. As of September 7, 2021: https://www.gao.gov/assets/gao-12-992.pdf

U.S. Government Accountability Office, *Defense Health Care: Actions Needed to Determine the Size and Readiness of Operational Medical and Dental Forces*, GAO-19-206, February 2019. As of September 6, 2021:
https://www.gao.gov/assets/gao-19-206.pdf

VA—*See* U.S. Department of Veterans Affairs.

Veterans Navigator, "Veterans Health Administration: Where Do I Get the Care I Need?" webpage, last updated May 3, 2021. As of November 19, 2022:
https://veteransnavigator.org/article/63525/veterans-health-administration

VHA Interagency Health Affairs, "DoD/VA Sharing Agreements," U.S. Department of Veterans Affairs and U.S. Department of Defense, briefing, undated. As of September 7, 2021:
https://rwtf.defense.gov/Portals/22/Documents/Meetings/m18/021dodva.pdf

Vought, Russell T., "Phase 1 Implementation of the Foundations for Evidence-Based Policymaking Act of 2018: Learning Agendas, Personnel, and Planning Guidance," Memorandum M-19-23, July 10, 2019. As of September 10, 2021:
https://www.whitehouse.gov/wp-content/uploads/2019/07/M-19-23.pdf

Walsh, Matthew M., Kevin A. Gluck, Glenn Gunzelmann, Tiffany Jastrzembski, and Michael Krusmark, "Evaluating the Theoretic Adequacy and Applied Potential of Computational Models of the Spacing Effect," *Cognitive Science*, Vol. 42, No. S3, 2018, pp. 644–691.

Walsh, Matthew M., and Marsha Lovett, "The Cognitive Science Approach to Learning and Memory," in Susan Chipman, ed., *The Oxford Handbook of Cognitive Science*, Oxford: Oxford University Press, 2016.

Weaver, Sallie J., David E. Newman-Toker, and Michael A. Rosen, "Reducing Cognitive Skill Decay and Diagnostic Error: Theory-Based Practices for Continuing Education in Health Care," *Journal of Continuing Education in the Health Professions*, Vol. 32, No. 4, 2012, pp. 269–278.

Westfall, Rebecca, "Tactical Combat Medical Care Course Hones Combat Medical Readiness," U.S. Army, May 6, 2019. As of September 7, 2021:
https://www.army.mil/article/220898/tactical_combat_medical_care_course_hones_combat_medical_readiness

Wiggins, Laura L., Janice Sarasnick, and Nathan G. Siemens, "Using Simulation to Train Medical Units for Deployment," *Military Medicine*, Vol. 185, Nos. 3–4, March 2, 2020, pp. 341–345.

Wisher, Robert, Mark Sabol, and John Ellis, *Staying Sharp: Retention of Military Knowledge and Skills*, U.S. Army Research Institute Special Report 39, July 1999. As of September 6, 2021:
https://apps.dtic.mil/sti/pdfs/ADA366825.pdf

W. K. Kellogg Foundation, *Logic Model Development Guide*, January 2004. As of September 13, 2021: https://www.wkkf.org/resource-directory/resources/2004/01/logic-model-development-guide

Xu, Yichi, Wenjing Xu, Aiyuan Wang, Haoye Meng, Yu Wang, Shuyun Liu, Rui Li, Shibi Lu, and Jiang Peng, "Diagnosis and Treatment of Traumatic Vascular Injury of Limbs in Military and Emergency Medicine: A Systematic Review," *Medicine*, Vol. 98, No. 18, May 2019, article e15406. As of September 25, 2021: https://doi.org/10.1097/MD.0000000000015406

Yau, Christopher W. H., Elena Pizzo, Steve Morris, David E. Odd, Cathy Winter, and Timothy J. Draycott, "The Cost of Local, Multi-Professional Obstetric Emergencies Training," *Acta Obstetricia et Gynecologica Scandinavica*, Vol. 95, No. 10, October 2016, pp. 1111–1119.

Young, Dwane, "99th MDG Seeks Trauma Accreditation," Defense Visual Information Distribution Service, July 31, 2020. As of September 7, 2021: https://www.dvidshub.net/news/375076/99th-mdg-seeks-trauma-accreditation

Zhang, Irene Y., Mark Thomas, Barclay T. Stewart, Eleanor Curtis, Carolyn Blayney, Samuel P. Mandell, Vance Y. Sohn, and Tam N. Pham, "Validation of a Low-Cost Simulation Strategy for Burn Escharotomy Training," *Injury*, Vol. 51, No. 9, September 2020, pp. 2059–2065.